LIVING OUT OF THE BOOK

Philip Hill

chipmunkapublishing
the mental health publisher
empowering people with schizophrenia

Philip Hill

Published by
Chipmunkapublishing
PO Box 6872
Brentwood
Essex CM13 1ZT
United Kingdom

http://www.chipmunkapublishing.com

Chipmunkapublishing gratefully acknowledges the support of Arts Council England.

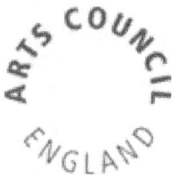

LIVING OUT OF THE BOOK

Introduction

Parts 3 to 7 written between 1994 and 1996 as part of 'Femme Fatale':

A Personal Experience of Schizophrenia.
Published by Auto-biographical Publications.
July, 1996.

Introduction Chapters 1, 2, 8, 9 and conclusion written between October 2005 and January 2008.

Philip Hill

Dedication

To Professor Marian Barnes and Professor Ann Davis whose intense input into my writing skills whilst writing my academic thesis has been a crucial part of my ability to put the 'chapters' of this auto biography together. Special thanks also to Moyra Riseborough who changed my thinking about disability issues.

Thanks to Disability Group "Tragic but Brave" for enabling me to believe I could work in social care. Thanks to Professor Femi Oyebode for giving me references for important jobs and student placements.

Philip Hill

LIVING OUT OF THE BOOK

TO ALL MY FAMILY – YOU KNOW WHO YOU ARE

Philip Hill

ACKOWLEDGEMENTS

Thanks to my twin brother for making some suggestions on redrafting for the chapters relating to my childhood. Thanks to Professor Ann Davis for her feedback on the first draft. My thanks also to my friend Mark Innes for his comments on numerous drafts. Thanks to Joanne Golding for typing up the previous incarnation of this book. Thanks to Linda Burden for enabling me to believe my life story could be of interest to others. Finally, thanks to my psychotherapist Maureen who inspired me to reflect on my own life as a way of moving on.

Cover photograph: Taken in 1970, in the garden of 110 Perry Wood Road, Perry Barr. The picture depicts me (on the right) and my twin brother in space suits within a Year of the Apollo Mission when Neil Armstrong first set foot on the moon.

Philip Hill

LIVING OUT OF THE BOOK

CONTENTS

FOREWORDS TO 1996 and 2008 editions –
By Professor Femi Oyebode
AUTHOR'S INTRODUCTION

CHAPTER 1
BECOMING A MAVERICK

CHAPTER 2
THE INEXPLICABLE EXPERIENCE THAT
BECAME LABELLED AS SCHIZOPHRENIA

PART 3
MY RELAPSE

PART 4
REHABILITATION

PART 5
EYE WITNESS ACCOUNTS OF MY ILLNESS

PART 6
MY QUEST TO FIND WORK

PART 7
MY EXPERIENCE AS A MENTAL HEALTH
CARER

CHAPTER 8
MY POSTGRADUATE JOURNEY

Philip Hill

CHAPTER 9
BEING A SOCIAL WORK STUDENT AND
BECOMING A SOCIAL WORKER

CONCLUSION

LIVING OUT OF THE BOOK

Foreword: Femi Oyebode MD., MRCPsych

Clinical Director: South Birmingham Mental Health Trust

Philip Hill has written a lucid and particularly human account of his experience of mental illness and of his rehabilitation. His determination and will, to gain control of his life in spite of the rupture which schizophrenia caused and which drug treatment was liable to perpetuate stand of an example of human dignity and courage in the face of difficult experiences. His book will, I believe, be of value to other sufferers and their families and there is no doubt that the professional careers will also benefit from reading it.

A personal account of this kind is especially important, as it demonstrates that whilst diseases such as schizophrenia inescapably affect the mind, there is yet a living, breathing being with the capacity for making judgments and for documenting the complexity of the experience of schizophrenia, at the core of the disease. This simple, but often forgotten, fact emphasizes the need to continue to treat individuals suffering from mental illness with respect and compassion. We should not need to be reminded about this but we live in an imperfect world and there is much stigma attached to persons with a history of mental illness.

Philip Hill

In Janet Frame's book 'Faces in the Water' when the heroin was discharged from hospital one of the nurses told her "when you leave hospital you must forget all that you have ever seen, put it out of your mind completely as if it never happened, and go live a normal life in the outside world". We should be grateful that Philip Hill has not heeded this kind of advice but instead has written an account which informs and inspires others.

LIVING OUT OF THE BOOK

Foreword to the second edition : Femi Oyebode MBBS, MD, PhD, FRCPsych, February 2008

Philip Hill has considerably expanded his autobiography. In the previous edition he concentrated on his experience of mental illness and rehabilitation. In the newly extended version we learn about Philip Hill's childhood, his education and progress through to university and his life since the irruption of schizophrenia in his young adulthood. We also learn about Philip Hill's family. I felt very privileged to have been invited to provide a foreword for the first edition. Reading this new edition, I feel inspired and humbled by Philip Hill's candour, his willingness to share his experiences with us, his capacity for reflection and his unswerving courage.

Lewis Wolpert in his book Malignant Sadness tells of how his wife was fearful that if the truth of his depression were to be widely known it would affect his career. When he recovered he wrote an article about his experience of depression in *The Guardian* newspaper and was surprised at the positive response but also on being complimented for being so brave. That was when he realized how much stigma there was still associated with depression. As with depression so it is with schizophrenia. There is still an unwarranted stigma associated with all forms of mental illness that to write about one's experience is still an act of courage. Philip Hill is doubly courageous. He has worked with tenacity to overcome the limits and restrictions which mental illness can impose on making a fruitful and successful life. And he has more than succeeded. He has also braved the inclement atmosphere, putting his professional progress at risk in order to speak to a wider audience about his experiences. That is a credit to him and a benefit to us all.

Philip Hill's book follows in the tradition of other writers who have gone on to describe their experiences of severe mental ilness, principally of psychosis. Perhaps the best known of these works are: John Perceval's *A Narrative of the treatment experienced by a gentleman during a state of derangement; Designed to explain the causes and the nature of insanity,* first published in 1840 and Daniel Schreber's *Memoirs of my mental illness*, published in 1903. Philip Hill's book, like these books, continues to stand before us as an example of the best of the human spirit. The sheer capacity to triumph in the face of adversity and to live to tell the tale is of itself admirable. And, being story-telling animals we admire even more the ability to tell the tale in a unique and interesting manner. Philip Hill's story is uplifting and inspiring. It is worthy of the attention it will get.

THE INTRODUCTION

The audience I am writing for.

I enter this book into the public arena with a bit of trepidation. After all when you describe, with blunt honesty, the logic of psychotic thought processes to a large audience you are not doing it to improve your image. What I am intending to do is give an understanding of the journey from sanity to insanity and back to those who are open minded enough to let their views and preconceptions about psychotic illness are challenged.

Furthermore I also intend to show that people with severe mental health issues can achieve at least some of their dreams if stigma, discrimination and prejudice of key 'gatekeeper's' can be overcome. In my life university tutors, my psychiatrist, occupational health departments of various employers have had the power over the extent to which I have been able to achieve my dreams.

It is easy to receive the negative signals from others and internalize them yourself. I have been lucky to have been someone who has believed in me and in my ongoing journey of recovery from mental health issues.

From my own experience and talking to others who have a similar diagnosis to me, I have come to the conclusion schizophrenia is one of the worst things you can be labeled with. People with our label are considered quite often as necessarily violent, irrational, eccentric and aggressive. When I see media representations of people diagnosed with schizophrenia I often feel I belong to an alien species or even worse that I do not belong at all. I find the occasions when people with our diagnosis are seen as an asset or particularly gifted are rare indeed. Books that put a positive slant on schizophrenia such as Peter Chadwick's "Schizophrenia: The Positive Perspective: In search of Dignity for Schizophrenic People' (1997). (Routeledge) are few and far between.

As a young child I was wrongly diagnosed with learning disabilities. The resulting stigma and discrimination caused me to be separated from my peer group at a crucial stage in my life and this was to have severe repercussions for my later personal development and may have contributed to my later mental health issues.

Stigma, prejudice and discrimination present barriers to full inclusion for mental health service users in society that are just as disabling, in my own opinion, as the symptoms of the illness and side effects of the medication they take. Over-protectiveness, institutionalized practices and stigma also prevent people with learning disabilities having full lives. Acknowledging the importance of these issues is an important part of how social workers are trained. However, this book is not just aimed at preaching to the easily converted such as social workers, approved social workers and social work students it is also aimed to challenge those from a medical background to broaden their value base so that models of intervention that build on service users strength are adopted rather than the deficit led approach that underpins much of the medical model. I have no doubt that this book could benefit learning disability nurses, psychiatric nursing students, student psychiatrists and even psychiatrists themselves. I do believe that my book could provide valuable case study material to psychology students.

As a social work professional (with adults with learning disabilities) I would expect to read autobiographical material to improve my understanding of other service users I come into contact with and I feel that other professionals need to do this for the sake of their own development. I believe disability narratives are one of many sources of information that nurses, doctors, consultants, social workers and occupational therapists can read to improve and inform their practice.

I feel that carers are often bombarded with medical explanations of mental illness when their relative becomes unwell. I believe that my book can provide a sense of hope that, while the road to recovery is long and full of setbacks, people with mental health issues can gain a sense of meaningful purpose to their lives in the long term if carers are careful not to reinforce negative perceptions that the person they care for may have of themselves. Recovery does not mean 'cure', it means that a person is able to cope with the worst aspects of their mental health issues on a day-to-day basis, whilst learning to contextualize this within a positive perception of themselves and be able to function at a level that gives them long-term fulfillment and a sense of purpose, meaning and hope to their lives.

The voluntary sector has a long established and growing involvement in supporting mental health service users on a day-to-day basis. Many non professional but highly skilled staff within the voluntary sector builds relationships with mental health service users based on mutual understanding and trust. Reading mental health survivor narratives can help reinforce and deepen understanding on which trust is built. Trust is a powerful tool when encouraging service users to engage (as someone who worked as a mental health rehabilitation worker in the voluntary sector for ten years I am allowed to say that).

My aim is not only to challenge but to provide a sense of hope to those with disabilities, particularly mental health survivors, that if you believe in yourself you can surprise people and achieve at least some of your dreams. The journey to achieve your dreams may be hard and the road traveled may be full of set backs but in the end expectations of many disabled people are often so low that even if we only get to a mid point on our destination we will have surprised many people, even those powerful professionals.

Personal reasons for writing this book

Seven years after my initial breakdown it was clear I had not moved on from the psychological issues that had initially disturbed me. It was then that I was referred for psychotherapy. In preparation for this talking therapy I wrote a four page explanation of the story behind my illness. It was then that a work colleague, Linda Burden, who had arranged to have the account typed up, suggested that my story may be of use to other people. I then elaborated on my story to produce a book called "Femme Fatale: A Personal Experience of Schizophrenia".

I then distributed copies of this book through a vanity publishing business called 'Autobiographical Publications'. I received much positive written and verbal feedback which made everything worthwhile. The most touching story was from a carer in the south Midlands who said that she had been unable to engage with her stepson for two decades. She claimed that after reading my book she was able to relate to him in a whole new way. Her last words were: thanks for giving my son back to me.

After selling about 300 copies of the first incarnation of this book, I then decided to put this mental health awareness project to rest.

Nine years later has my fortieth birthday party approached I had a bit of an existential crisis. What had I really achieved in my life? Was I really destined to be a social worker for the rest of my life? Was I ever going to be famous? What would people say my contribution was when I was dead? My life seemed mapped out before me. My feelings were intensified because I had been unable to attain my doctorate, getting the consolation prize of an MPhil research degree instead. This apparent failure had put my ambitions for an academic career on hold. The feelings that I had at this time are best described in a chapter called The Emotional and Social Development in Middle Adulthood in "Development Through the Lifespan' (2001, 2nd edition, AlLynn and Bacon) by Laura E Berk, page 525.

Around forty people evaluate their success in meeting early adulthood goals. Realizing that from now on more time will lie behind than ahead, they regard the remaining years as increasingly precious...........Whether these years bring a gust of wind or a storm, most people turn inward for a time, focusing on personally meaningful living........... They ask, Can I still achieve what I wanted? If now, can I accept what I have attained? Even people who have reached their goals ask, what good are these accomplishments to other people, to society or to me?

I went to my psychiatrist with these issues and he said he could either refer me for therapy or I could write my autobiography, which would achieve much the same positive objectives without the need for a therapist.

When revisiting the earlier version of my autobiography, written from the perspective of a 30 year old, I felt that the fresh and spontaneous writing style of the 'Parts' that described my illness and its immediate aftermath could not be improved on. I therefore kept the 'Parts' 3, 4, 5, 6 and 7 and added 'Chapters' . I rewrote material that related to my childhood and undergraduate years to form (Chapter 1) and added an update of 2 chapters, on my postgraduate education (Chapter 8), and my experience of training and then becoming a social worker (Chapter 9).

As a thirty- year old man writing in the mid-90's I defined myself and my life story in terms of my illness. I was not ashamed to use the term schizophrenia to promote my book and felt it was okay to be referred to as a schizophrenic. Indeed I was very aware of the box office draw of using schizophrenia in the title of the book itself.

When writing as a man approaching forty years of age almost ten years later, I realized I had to some extent achieved a good deal more. I was now a professional social worker, a trained academic researcher and someone with over ten years experience of working within a professional capacity with fellow mental health survivors. I felt that in defining myself I was so much more than my illness and that I had underestimated the effect of being misdiagnosed as someone with learning disabilities on my late personal, social and emotional development that affects me to the present day.

When renaming this edition of my autobiography I wanted something that represented my spectacular, traumatic, yet unbalanced early development but also had a subtitle that described my journey to the person that I am happy to be today. The perseverance of my father in teaching me to read and the importance of books in my early life gave me a passport to escape a learning disabilities label but was only the beginning of a journey to achieving social and emotional milestones at a delayed pace. The rupture that schizophrenia and anti-psychotic medication cause me led to further delays in my personal development.

The acceptance of fellow mental health survivors finally gave me a peer group in which I could feel a sense of belonging. It now matters that I conform and that I fit in, I am no longer trying to be different to everyone else.

I hope you fine this book enjoyable and challenging.
January 29th, 2008.

P.S. Some of the names of people in this book have been changed to protect the identities of certain individuals.

CHAPTER ONE

BECOMING A MAVERICK:

MY JOURNEY FROM A DIAGNOSIS OF A LEARNING DISABILITY TO LIFE AT UNIVERSITY.

I was told later in my life that I had been neglected in a children's home with nothing to compensate for the bonding that should have taken place with my natural mother from whom I was separated at birth. By the time I was told that the person who I thought of as my mother was in fact my foster mother I was about nine. My foster mother had always said that I had two mothers but I did not understand this until I was nine. It was about that time that I understood why Mr. Mason visited every six months. I found out that he was a children's social worker.

All I comprehended in the early 1970's living in Perry Barr was that when I played with my brother Paul in Perry Wood Road was that we were both rejected by the neighboring children. "You go to that school where all the Mongols go" was the exact phrase they kept repeating to us.

I was later to find out that I was an outcast in the eyes of my neighbors because I shared my friendship at Amblecote special school with children some of whom had Down's syndrome. That led to me being labeled different from an early age by my peers. I was about nine when I realized I was in a special school for children with learning disabilities but it was to be another couple of years before I was to grasp why I had been placed there at the age of five.

The official labeling process started when my brother and I failed to integrate into Perry Beeches, an infant mainstream school. An assessment by a child psychologist followed. His assessment was that we would need to be placed in a school for our special educational needs. The best my parents could hope for was that both of us would progress from special school to the bottom of a mainstream school.

I did not grasp that I was in a special school but I noticed that my brother used to copy the facial presentations of his classmates with Down's syndrome. My foster mother, Jessica shouted at him and told him not to copy the expressions of his classmates. "If you keep doing that you'll stick like it", she said.

The whole world changed for me when after a Sunday evening when I saw my foster father Albert play in a band called Fiesta. The whole evening was pretty stimulating and I ended up doing what a lot of children of that age like doing, which is stopping up late. The next day at school I drew two men with guitars, my dad on saxophone, someone else on drums and the lead singer with a microphone. I was asked questions about this picture by my form teacher. I explained it was my dad's band, named all the instruments and before I knew it I was summoned to the headmistress. Rather than being in trouble I was told that I had got the best work award. Within a short amount of time the headmistress was to meet my parents. She said that my parent's assertion that I was ready to go to main school was something she had initially disagreed with but now she had to admit they had been right. As my foster mother Jessica said "They find it so easy to stick you in these places but it's bloody hard to get you out".

Any notion that I would be allowed to stay in the comfort zone of the bottom stream of mainstream primary school was soon dispelled when my foster father, Albert said it was unacceptable that I still could not read. He was quite directive and initially angry at my lack of motivation. My foster mother, Jessica had tried to teach me to read but I was very sensitive to the emotion expressed in her voice when my progress slowed. Albert taught me as though time was of the essence. Within six months which effectively meant my tenth birthday, I could read my dad's *Sun* newspaper. I found it difficult to understand how he could teach me to read whilst driving his Ford Cortina Mark Two while I sat in the long plastic seating in the back. An example of how much I had progressed was the fact that within 12 months I progressed through twenty books of the Peter and Jane series. However, what captured my imagination when learning to read was the pirate series. The main characters were Captain Red, who wore ruby jewels and Captain Blue who wore sapphire jewels.

Albert had a very basic approach to education. If you want to find out anything all you needed to know was how to find the right book about it in the library and devote the time to studying it. I was to find out years later that Albert had started a job as a draughtsman without qualifications on how to design electrical switchgear. He was scared of faking it and being found out so he borrowed a book from the library and laid out the living room with cotton reels as transistors, cups as resistors and so on and then played out different scenarios from the book on how the circuit would behave in different circumstances. I think my dad overdid it a bit as before long he was promoted to senior z\draughtsman and then chief draughtsman.

Being in a household where my foster mother had high standards of tidiness meant that reading was one of the more acceptable activities in which I could engage myself without making too much mess. My first reading project was inspired by the then headmaster of Audley Junior School who instilled the notion of courage in a talk in assembly. The role model and very embodiment of courage in his opinion was Admiral Lord Nelson. My image of Nelson was of the black guy who I had known at special school who had bullied me. So when I visited Glebe Farm library and opened the pages of my first history book I was extremely surprised that Nelson was white. I found it difficult to focus on the blocks of text in the book but built up my knowledge by reading the subscripts to each illustration. What little knowledge I had I seemed to wear on my sleeve and was unbearably big headed about it all. This did not stop my mom boasting to neighbours that I had a photographic memory. It is true that I knew the technique of how to memorize things but only things I was motivated to remember. I seemed to forget to wipe my shoes on the carpet before entering the kitchen and always seemed to forget to empty my pockets before putting my clothes in for washing. In many ways I seemed to be a scatter brain on issues that mattered to my mom. Unlike my brother I never volunteered for any household chores.

My foster mother made a contribution to my life because of the gifts she has given me. The gifts bought by my parents such as the Airfix model of the HMS Victory, the Lone Ranger action figure on horseback and the Hutchinson Encyclopedia lose their significance over the years. What remains are the gifts my mom gave me in terms of her long term influence on my character. Because she was around a great deal more than my foster father she was the most important adult role model in my life when I was growing up. The adoptions of the most important aspects of her approach to life have been a good foundation stone for adulthood. I inherited two important moral values from mum. Firstly, she taught me that honesty in life is the best policy otherwise you always get found out in the end. She also taught me the value of hard work even if you fail at least you can say you tried your best. I used to annoy my mother when I was young because I was absent minded. This was something I always tried to rectify but seemed powerless to change. I was never as thoughtful or considerate as my twin brother being prone to be full of my own importance. My fear is that those early impressions have left a long term image to her of who I still am when in fact I moved on a great deal in terms of who I am and what is important to me. I remember trying to please my mother as a young child but never being able despite trying to rectify the faults she saw in me.

Our mum used to often let off steam at us on Sunday afternoons. Whilst doing the ironing she would say things like none of us are perfect, we all do things wrong and said everyone had their faults. She said to me that I would probably always be untidy and that there was nothing she could do about that, that's just who you are she would say. After sessions like these my brother and I would always feel like we had had a psychological lift.

Although I have always striven to be honest in life as a way of taking on board my mums approach to life I have always struggled to be honest about my feelings. Knowing how you feel involves taking yourself away from a place where you are considering how others may view the choices you make in life. In my opinion you need to have had a childhood in which you were able to disagree with your parents and express those views without fear. That involves being brave and being prepared to be ridiculed and criticized and labeled as naughty in the process. My lack of courage in challenging my parents and being prepared to disagree with them contrasts with my sister. Lynne wasn't prepared to accept the quiet life but was always pushing the boundaries knowing full well she might have to face the undesirable consequences such as being grounded or told to go to her room. There were many times I saw her cry wishing I could cry too but being afraid to show my emotions. The difference between me and my sister was that she was prepared to take the risks and fall out with her parents and I wasn't. Because my sister chose the difficult path in childhood I feel she probably did not go through the identity crisis I was to go through at university. Avoiding doubts about who you are, involves knowing how you feel and being able to express this. Isolated from friends and suppressing my own feelings to please my parents, my childhood was a lonely experience accompanied only by the support of my family with no wider social circle.

Mornings between 7.40 and 8.00am were normally the periods of quality time that I spent on my own with my foster father. These periods were normally times when my dad reviewed the previous nights Villa game to me or when I asked questions like how big is the Universe and what happens when you die. My dad was not hesitant in offering his philosophy to these complex questions. He came up with gems like the weather always evens itself out in the long run and when you are an adult no-one notices when you are doing your job but everyone notices when you are not. Knowing the line up of the early and mid-1970's Villa team was a good way to get into my dads good books as well as a weekly opportunity to develop my memory skills. Let's check that team photo again. Jim Combes in goal, Brian Geoffrey, Willie Anderson, Chico Hamilton, John Robson' Ray Graydon, Andy Lockhead, Brian little, Bruce Ricoh and manager Viv Crowe. Aston Villa were then in the third division and my first home game was seeing Villa against Cardiff City around 1971-1972 season. I do not know how he did it but he held both me and my brother on his shoulder while we watched the game. My developing specialist knowledge was supplemented by keeping a scrapbook.

My dad was prone to the odd moment of madness when screaming and shouting at the slightest excuse. This happened when Ray Graydon scored a rebound from a penalty to win the League cup against Norwich City in 1975 or when Brian little scored from an acute angle to win the League cup against Everton in 1977. Nothing ever tops the time when Villa were playing on a live television broadcast from Rotterdam. My dad was playing solitaire with the television on in the background. Tony Morley interrupted my dad's concentration. My dad looked up at the TV in response to the commentators raised voice when Morley ran a Bayer Munich defender inside out and crossed the ball so that Peter With almost missed from point blank range as the ball went in from the inside of the left hand post. My dad instantaneously threw the cards in the air and screamed momentarily and ran to kiss and hug my mother as she was peeling potatoes at the sink. That night Villa was crowned champions of Europe.

My dad was short of money for a long period of time between 1975 and 1978 when working for a small business. His pay cheques kept bouncing and I often felt guilty about asking him for pocket money at this time. Though money was tight at home when it came round to the annual holiday to Dorset no expense was spared as I lavished spending from pocket money I had been encouraged to save all year. The usual diet was abandoned because it was a chip supper every night.

In December 1974 I met my foster sister Lynn as a two-month old baby. She lay there content with what I remember to be a small growth of hair. Over the next nine years, before I went to university I was to witness every stage of her development from the perspective of being nine-and-a-half years older than her. It is true and fair to say that my parents were more lenient in the way they brought Lynn up than they were in the way they brought up my brother and me.

My mum used to explain this by saying that when my brother and I were young she had to go through a lot of hurdles to earn her right to become our mother. Regular visits from health professionals, social workers and constant attendance at clinics meant she was always peering over her shoulders on how her parenting appeared to a larger audience. Our special school background and the rejection we experienced from children our own age made us in her opinion more vulnerable. As a result she was more protective of my brother and me than she needed to be with Lynn.

My brother and I were both teased by Lynn. I chose to ignore a great deal of the teasing and Lynn soon gave up on winding me up. However, my brother Paul always seemed to rise to the bait and got himself into trouble. I always felt that my sister respected and trusted me as we grew up. However, one day I felt I abused that trust. She came home from school telling me that her teacher had told her that God created the world. Rather than thinking and engaging my brain I tried to undermine everything she said. I have learned through experience just how tough life is and in my opinion what people need to survive is hope. Whatever the source where people find hope is not a matter for me to judge. One day someone may prove there is no supernatural being in the Universe, however, that does not deny that for millions of people a mere belief in God is a source of hope and a way of coping. There is no excuse for taking a source of hope away from anyone in my opinion. If my sister gets to read this I hope she will understand what I mean.

At one stage it could have been argued that Lynn may have grown up without the necessity of discipline. However, I feel Lynn was allowed to act out the child role to a complete extent and develop in a very natural way into the sensitive, fun loving and caring mother she is now. It has taken me longer to reach adulthood than my sister because I was more ambitious academically. Other sides to my personal development were therefore somewhat delayed. I had no social circle outside the family or outside of school. My parents had tried to send us to a church youth group, Sunday school and Scouts. However, we struggled to fit in with the others and when we said we no longer wanted to go and our parents respected that decision.

I was so insecure when I started at Sir Wilfred Martineau Secondary School that I was petrified I could not cope with the pace of teaching at such a seemingly prestigious school. I followed my friend into the class because I thought the bottom stream class was mine. I was corrected and sent to Mrs. Poore's middle stream class which made me more anxious about my ability to cope at such a high level.

LIVING OUT OF THE BOOK

I had problems settling in, courtesy of my classmate Sean Brown who kept stealing things from me. My brother was later to work with Sean in a warehouse where he was caught stealing (no change there then).

In terms of social development there were a number of setbacks. Once again my brother Paul and I were rejected by neighbouring children once we had moved to Mears Drive, Stetchford. After a couple of years of trying to fit in with other children in the drive we once again retreated to the comfort zone indoors. At secondary school I would find it again difficult to fit in and make friends easily. The people I found it easiest to mix with were fellow victims of bullying. I found my best friend in the world was my brother, everything else seemed at a superficial level. In my third year at Sir Wilfred Martineau School my form teacher Miss Turner expressed concerns about my social development to my parents. These were concerns which in effect I feel should have rung alarm bells with my parents. Instead, I continued my one dimensional academic development.

Not only did I lack social skills but in many ways I was anti social. Feeling a need to achieve on the physical education front I had resorted to running to school each morning with a haversack on my back. I was dubbed by fellow pupils as "Steve Austin the Six Million Dollar Man", a well-known character on television in the mid-1970. This was because I raced the number 14 bus over the two mile route to school overtaking the bus when it stopped to pick up pupils. They used to sing the theme tune to me as I ran past the bus stop. Unwittingly I had turned myself from outcast to a freak show. Mr. Hall the physical education teacher said to me once, referring to my lack of personal hygiene "You dirty, dirty man".

There were paybacks though to my daily training ritual. I finally achieved my first sporting success by winning the 1500 meters on sports day beating a good sporting all rounder Michael Griffin in the home straight in a sprint finish. On the cross country front I was second three years in a row to the schools sporting 'Good at Everything' Anthony Andrew's, finally running him into the ground when I won the cross country in the sixth form championships. I did achieve recognition for this improvement in my physical shape being selected to be part of the schools athletics team and by winning a certificate on school prize day for progress in physical education. However, physically I looked like a geek. I had what looked like a match stick like body and it was another ten years in my mid-twenties before I filled out at all.

After a couple of years of finishing towards the top of my class on the exam front I was promoted to the top stream at school. In effect this meant that I was expected to get a string of 'O' Levels in my final exams.

By the time of the fourth year in the top stream I had managed to escape the bully and his gang. This I had managed to do by no longer having to do physical education in which I was seen as some underweight geek who couldn't achieve anything. I had also managed to ensure that I was indoors during lunch and morning breaks by becoming a librarian.

I had a pretty creepy way of vainly trying to ensure that I had an easy ride at the expense of my twin brother. I honestly believed I was better than my brother but the sibling rivalry reached such a pitch that on reflection I probably derived a great deal of pleasure from getting him into trouble. I thrived on opportunities to tell tales on him and to join the wholesale criticism that was directed at him. True, my brother's antics could be seen as challenging in the mild sense of the word, however, he was my best friend and you don't grass on a friend.

Purposefully getting my brother into trouble was a way of earning Brownie points with mum and dad and steering their critical gaze away from me. I do not understand to this day how my brother tolerated my behavior. I feel bad now about undermining his relationship with mum and dad and destroying his confidence at a critical point in his life. My parents and Nan were pivotal in enabling me to adopt a better attitude to my brother in the early 1990's. I feel that the behavior of many people including myself, fellow school pupils and later his work colleagues who poked fun at his difference, were in a way responsible for a process that was to eventually undermine his mental health. Mum used to say that my brother had a persecution complex and always felt people were against him, I feel I played a crucial role in turning mum and dad against my brother. It's too late to repair the damage now but I will do whatever I can no matter how long it takes to build my brother up again.

Paul was judged as ready to leave Special School at the age of twelve. Knowing the type of rough school Alderlea Boys had become I decided I needed to give Paul advice about his walking posture. He had a very effeminate walking style. If he persisted in his walking posture I knew he would be beaten up at school. I displayed to him a more conspicuous walking style more akin to a casual march. To this day Paul walks in the way I taught him but still has the discretion to camp it up when he wants.

My brother decided to 'come out' in 1992. He struggled to find a way to tell the family and I remember my dad being outraged by the seemingly insensitive my brother revealed his sexuality to him on the phone. We were all shocked but I feel it took a while for other members of the family to accept my brother really was gay. However, despite being shocked myself I immediately accepted what my brother said about his feelings as factual. In the weeks that followed I felt Paul had been very brave to disclose in the manner he had. It felt to me he was finally taking control over who he was and how he wanted others to perceive him. Leaving home at 22 had clearly been the right time so that he fully understood the need to disclose in his mid-twenties on his own terms.

Paul accompanied me on fortnightly visits to the library in Ward End in the late seventies and early eighties. Dad was always a good person to discuss my reading choices. He handed down to me some very old editions of 'Biggles' by Captain W.E. Johns, a battered 'Wind in the Willows' and his extensive collection of James Bond novels in the originally published sixties Pan paperback editions. Initially I reveled in 'Alice's Adventures in Wonderland' as an 11 year old. I kept wondering whether I would ever encounter anyone in my life like the Queen of Hearts. I always found the meticulous preparations of Enid Blyton's 'Famous Five' pretty exciting, particularly the 'Fives' fascination with pilchard sandwiches. However, during my teens my tendency was to get fiction that was a bit too old for my understanding of life and I wondered why I had problems grasping more than a literal interpretation of what I had read. Books like 'Tom Brown's Schooldays' and 'David Copperfield' were difficult for me to concentrate on because in addition to a more sophisticated writing style there were endless blocks of text containing lots of characters weaving in a complex way in and out of the main plot. My memory was always good but my concentration was abysmal, a situation that was to reverse twenty-five years later as a mature student. At least with a non fiction book you could dip in and out of the text and grasp a great deal from the explanation of diagrams, tables, illustrations and charts. I always had problems in concentrating because of my own short attention span and the noisy nature of the house especially with the radio always on.

My mum and Nan were concerned that I was spending most of my time reading factual books and felt I should be reading more fiction. This they said was a more usual way that children read. However, I largely ignored their advice.

My favorite present as a child of thirteen was a 'Hutchinson's Encyclopedia' a massive one volume edition. You could read this book and dip in-and-out of it without much concentration required and yet you could build up quite massive amounts of knowledge quite quickly without much effort. Such knowledge was useful when watching Nicholas Parson's 'Sale of the Century', Jimmy Tarbuck's 'Winner Takes All' and the general knowledge quiz of 'Mastermind'. Furthermore, I made a healthy contribution to the Sunday Express General Knowledge Prize Crossword, a ritual family event after Sunday lunch.

As a librarian at school I had regular access to their 22-volume Encyclopedia. As a child in my early teens any spare time I could get to study this wonderful book was pure Heaven.

I developed an encyclopedic knowledge of British Naval History, British political history, especially monarchy, a basic grasp of evolution from an old book and David Attenborough's 'Life on Earth' TV series and a rudimentary knowledge of geography from the Atlas I had been bought one Christmas. However, the Holy Grail of Atlases was an historical atlas which gave me a visual representation of the territory fought over different periods of history. In particular I reveled in turn of the century maps of the British Empire at its greatest extent in about 1900. However, it was fascinating to discover how much the political map of Britain changed over the course of the English Civil War. My initial encounter with British History in primary school was through the illustrated R.J. Unstead children's books. Again I found it difficult to concentrate on blocks of text for any period but found the subscripts to the illustrations useful to build up layers of knowledge.

As a way of developing my interest in Physics I tried to analyse diagrams describing different trains with a passenger carrying clocks whilst traveling at or close to the speed of light but even then I never quite grasped Einstein's General theory of Relativity.

Being a loner, reading was not the only solitary activity I spent my time engaged in. I was an avid stamp collector to the extent that I knew as much about stamps as some train spotter's know about trains. On reflection, I feel I had withdrawn myself over a number of years into my own solitary world and in a sense, my own reality.

My initial career choice was to become an engineering officer in the Royal Navy and my choice of study options in my third year reflected a heavy bias towards the sciences (Physics and Chemistry), Math's and English as core subjects, Metalwork, Technical Drawing, Geography and an indulgence in Economic and Social History of the British Isles.

My parents were both told by my Chemistry teacher Mr. Keating that I was not studying hard enough. No one wanted to study Chemistry in their spare time because Mr. Keating made the subject incomprehensible. "Mr. Keating cannot teach' was the 'in' phrase on the graffiti scrawled across exercise books. Nevertheless, Mr. Keating's comment from a late 1970's parents evening was to lead to the riot act being laid down by mum and dad. Being sensitive to and respectful of my parents I started a life long journey of self motivated study. I felt I had realized that a couple of years work could get me the job I wanted. How wrong I proved to be. I was nearly forty-years old before being anywhere near fulfilled in a job and greatly surprised at how much more study, sacrifice and setbacks I would eventually have to overcome to arrive at a very different destination to an armed forces career.

Furthermore, my limited progress in Math's was a potential threat to study science or engineering at anything more than a basic level. Failure to continue at 'A' Level Physics beyond a term was symptomatic of this. This took me a few years to get over. Staying on a year had resulted in getting an English 'O' Level but little else to add to the other four 'O' Levels and equivalent I had attained in the previous year.

My experience of education did cause me to challenge my parents in their views. The only issue I remember standing up to my foster parents about was the issue of race. At Hall Green College I had begun to make friends with peers my own age who were Asian and Afro-Caribbean. My parents still kept repeating their views that the ethnic minorities were taking over. They would always prefix what they said with 'I'm not a racist but.....' and would utter a statement about Asian people ruining this country. I disagreed with them a number of times until a time when my foster mother would come out with the usual views and then turn to me and say 'We know what you think'.

However, in 1999 I had a somewhat interesting discussion with my dad about Mohammed Ali's nomination for BBC Sports Personality of the Millennium'. He said he had changed his views on the nature of racism since moving up to Scotland.

A newspaper headline about a young English pupil in Scotland being beaten to death by Scottish pupils had made him realize how racism operated in his new adopted country and that he was now the outsider.

In the summer of 1979, after a family quarrel my brother and I were told where my natural mother lived. I had unwittingly met my mother before, not recognizing her (she was not introduced to me either). I remembered her as a ten year old boy – this strange and weird woman who wanted to cut a huge slice of her winter coat to bring it down to size.

When my brother and I knocked on the door of Alpha House in Hockley and asked to see Iris Hill, she came to the door gazed at us and broke into tears. She hardly said a word for the next hour as she sat with us, very tearful. Not being good at that age at understanding human feelings in this point of my life I found it difficult to explain to myself why my mother had cried. Over the coming years I was to understand that my mother spent most of the early and mid-1970s begging on the streets as a homeless person. My mother had had a breakdown at the age of twenty-two. Although she was not homeless now my mother needed the supervision of care staff around the clock to manage her so-called condition. My mother had a medical diagnosis of schizophrenia. Iris's husband, John Patrick Hill had left her just before we were born in the mid-1960s and nobody has seen anything of him since. He had apparently been a docker who had come from Liverpool and may well have been Irish. It was thought he may have returned to his home city.

When trying to draw the strands in the chapter about my childhood together there are a few things it is important to be explicit about. Without the intervention of my foster parents my brother and I would have been left to stagnate in that Pipe Hayes children's home, condemned to a life being labeled with a leaning difficulty. There may have been aspects of my childhood that have not been ideal but there are few people that survive their time with parents without some sort of baggage. I am disappointed that I did not achieve what I have in adult life earlier because it would have been a more fitting reward for the commitment, effort and sacrifices that had been made on my behalf by both mum and dad. Despite the fact that I have never met my biological father, my foster father is my only dad in my eyes. Furthermore, even though I built strong emotional bonds with my natural mother before she died my stronger emotional ties are with mum, my foster mother. Parenthood is difficult and costly in terms of sacrifices, time and energy. I do not feel I would ever be as good a parent as my parents were to me.

I was however to put both my parents, my brother and sister through a more difficult time before they could feel assured that I had made a transition to some of the trappings of adult life such as financial independence and a steady, secure job. Even though educationally I had caught up with my peers I needed to negotiate further psychological and emotional development milestones before I could relate to people my own age with ease. These were experiences that were to push me well outside my comfort zone and begin a very long journey towards maturity.

My preparation for living away from home in Leicester was in many respects inadequate for the difficult challenges ahead. A business studies diploma, the basis of selection for University was not steeped in enough academic rigour to help me with the 3000 word essays I was to face in the first weeks of the autumn semester. I understood a little about Economics the subject for which I was to study, but had not studied it to a sufficiently high level to help with its basic mathematical applications. I did not have experience of looking after myself for any substantial period before University. Despite efforts to make friends I was still seen as different everyone else at college. This was partly because I did not have a feel for fashion and did not venture outside of the friendship I made with Keith. Keith brought me out of my shell a bit and was always saying that I lacked confidence. The one thing I was always grateful to Keith for was teaching me how to play snooker. He played host on regular Saturday evenings when I played on his table and watched William Shatner in the cop series T.J. Hooker. I mixed with other people at college but did not keep contact outside college. I almost gave up college for a job at a Motor Insurance Company but the job offer never came and I ended up registering for my second year. It was the law lecturer who encourages some of our class to apply to the University Clearing Body for an Economics course. I decided to put Leicester as my first choice because it was far enough from home to gain some independence but close enough to go back if anything went wrong.

I remember my mum crying on the day she and dad dropped me off at Villiers Hall on my first day at Leicester University. It was one of the occasional moments when I was forced to realize how much I am really loved by my parents.

It did not take long to realize how hard I would still find it to make friends in Villiers Hall. I lived on the edge of the site in Treroose House. Traditionally this had been a place where they had placed working class Christians. I was a waverer at the time and other students when I told them where I lived asked if I was a Christian.

I tended to come straight home from lectures and go to play amongst a queue of people on the half-size snooker table in one of the old houses on site. What few close friends I had tended to hang about there. I remember a shop selling me a bent cue and finding out the hard way it was inappropriate to use on the table. The maximum break I ever achieved was 32.

Other students at Villiers set themselves challenges such as how many dry Weetabix you could eat in a single sitting. The winner found after almost wanting to vomit he could manage 21.

Then there was the JCR (Junior Common Room) committee and its yearly elections for a hall president. One candidate failed to do a speech but instead prepared for the predictable questions using a tape recorder to spool backwards or forwards to the appropriate lyrics or so he thought relevant from Queen Songs.

We had a pinball machine by the dining room which repeated a phrase like 'Try harder next time' if you did not get top score. One day our resident 'Mr. Angry' became drunk and played this machine. This time when the machine told him to try harder the glass got a bit smashed shall we say?

Then there was the Villiers Hall annual golden penis award. The winner received a glowing candle in the form of a waxed shaped penis with a wick which had been lighted. I came third in the race, my friend Gerard came second and a guy who was the accident prone bar manager who failed to get through a week or two without breaking some bone or other in his body won the prestigious award.

There was one student block where, no matter how they changed the selection policy there was always shall we say challenging behavior. As one student put it "How do they manage to put a complete bunch of assholes in Wighton (block) every single year?" I ventured to enter this hall one day and found rotting empty Chinese food cartons strewn around the rooms' downstairs, crushed, empty cans of Redstripe Lager and an assortment that can only be described as litter. I had heard the block had had a bit of a party and had managed to smash a few windows and let go of the odd fire extinguisher or two. However, before the hall warden could go round and inspect, fining them for the damage they had caused, the Wighton students realized it was cheaper to get a contract from Yellow Pages to fix everything up.

Despite fun times my first year was a struggle in terms of making and keeping friends. It became apparent just how hard it would be to build bridges with those with whom I lived after a night out with four people from Treroose. It was difficult to join in conversation at the right time with something that was relevant to the prevailing topic of conversation and I ended up being ridiculed by one student. After that I swapped rooms and moved in with someone who was even more of f loner than me. Duncan was a nice, polite and quiet person but he never ventured out of his room outside lectures. I felt really sorry for him. The problem with our room was that the window never opened which meant that my running kit could be smelt down the corridor between washes. Indeed I was not able to fully grasp the personal hygiene problems I had until nearly the end of the first year during which I managed to alienate everyone apart from a close group of loyal friends. Three of my best friends were Dave Jackson, Gerald Bane and Simon Pritchard. Gerard who preferred to be known by a left wing alias of Lev Jashin was a vegetarian, anarchist, self proclaimed White Rasta and collector of Reggae records. His famous assertion to fellow students was that the problem with vegetarian food was all that he was offered to eat was vegetables. My gaffe was almost as good. When asked whether I had a bike I said "No but I've got a chopper".

Dave was a music connoisseur and listened to John Peel religiously. His weak spot was that he could not get through his yearly summer exams without an overload of the Abba back catalogue. He only needed a three week course of treatment however to maintain his sanity which you need to do when you are studying a subject as hard as degree level physics. He tried to convert me to groups such as the 'Shop Assistants', 'Blue Aeroplane' and 'Working Week' unsuccessfully. Dave died in an accident at Ipswich Docks in 1990 and I lost someone who maintained loyalty to me when I struggled to keep friends with nearly everyone else, and he was a key figure in enabling me to maintain and keep my sanity for as long as I did. I tried to capture what David meant to me when I wrote to his grieving parents and three months later they sent me a letter back thanking me for my trouble.

Simon was a community activist who, as a member of the University Young Liberals was key in getting me to join this group because I was a member of the SDP (The Slowly Disappearing Party) at the time. Simon had had problems fitting into College Hall basically because he was different. He did not feel a need to conform to fashion and was in a way a shy person. What mattered to him was his faith, he was a Quaker (very untrendy) and the fact that he was passionate about politics (it was not trendy to be a Liberal either). Simon campaigned to get more litter bins in Knighton only to find that allegedly students set fire to them.

The gang of Liberals was managed by Jeff, (I can't remember his surname) and Rob Reynolds (now Lord Reynolds a Liberal sitting in the House of Lords). Other members were Matthew Jones (a fellow Economics Undergraduate eventually becoming a Transport Economist), Lorraine Groom (fellow Economics Undergraduate), Dave Jackson and Gerard Bane. We distributed 'Focus' leaflets and even stood as council candidates in unwinable seats. However, we were successful in taking one seat from Labour in Crown Hills and one seat from the Conservatives in Knighton. Reynolds had masterminded the Liberal bid to control Liverpool Council in 1979 and now he was trying to undermine Labour dominance in

Leicester. In the General Election Campaign of 1987 Leicester south was the most marginal seat in the country with a majority of seven for the Conservative MP Derek Spencer. In that year I lived in a flat at Elms Road student residences with right wing Monday Club members of the Conservative Party who did not take me very seriously until I had done canvassing in our local residences and Liberal posters started appearing everywhere. There was such a media spotlight on Leicester south that the Labour Party's 'Red Wedge' (a posse of pop stars of the time which included Jimmy Sommerville and Paul Weller) visited Leicester University on election eve to give a free concert.

The other University Societies I was a member of were the Athletics and Cross Country societies. Key characters I was to get to know were Plod, Sheep Turd, Barney, Frankie, Stu, Debbie and Rosie of those that I can remember. Weekends were often about racing in a running event that often involved travel, physical exertion then beer. Typical pranks were to turn up at McDonald's (or as we knew it McBurger's) at five-to-eleven (P.M.) and order a Big Mac meal for ten to eat in. Another thing was to go to Pizza Hut and stack so much self service side salad on our plates it collapsed in a heap on the table. The Cross Country Society blew the total expenses budget in a single weekend in Glasgow at the BUSF Championships. What do you expect though when you book into a five-star hotel? The race was followed by a late night version of what has become the tradition that is known as the Chunder Mile. Sheep Turd decided he would participate and race someone from Leeds University. They both stripped off and it was pouring with rain. The rule was that the mile was to consist of four 400 metre laps and after each 400 metres there was the requirement to drink a pint of beer. It is highly likely that such exertions would cause the participant to vomit after two to three laps, hence the word chunder.

Our athletics coach was Dave (Dave the ball breaker). One of his more typical sessions was ten repetitions of 400 metres with 90-second jog recovery – and we hated him for it. To add insult to injury he tried to flog membership of the gym he had just set up.

There was no room for elitism in our sports clubs, such notions could be entertained by top Universities such as Birmingham Loughborough. There is a story that Loughborough turned up to one race in anticipation of winning by bringing a number of bottles of Champagne with them. As far as Leicester University was concerned the better runners in the A Team Road Relay team would run a second leg for the B Team to enable less able runners a chance to run. This type of consideration for other runners was not strictly within the rules. So runners running a second leg would make up pseudo-names such as P. Lod, C.

Birdseye, P. Llonker and so on. None of the officials I hasten to add caught on.

Being a member of the Athletics and Cross Country Club was a good way to get round the country. Autumn involved going to London for the UCLA Cross Country Relays at Parliament Hill. Spring meant a trip up north for the Durham University Road Relays then back to London for Hyde Park Road Relays followed by trips to Athletic Stadiums such as Meadow bank in Edinburgh and Crystal Palace. I remember that in my final year I gradually set about beating nearly all of my team mates in one race or another. I ran ten kilometers (just over six miles) in little over 31 and-a-half minutes, and 5km in 15 minutes & 30-seconds and 800 metres in 2 minutes & 3-seconds.

I had a very task orientated approach to life at University. This was partly derived from the way my mum used to juggle her responsibilities. I remember her organizing her day by ticking off tasks one-by-one on a huge list. She constantly felt the need to check things over-and-over again to ensure she had not forgotten anything. My brother's reaction to this was to put the same amount of effort into the detail of the way he did things as she did. When experiencing my first taste of independence I became almost allergic to detail. Getting things done was important even if the quality of what I did was not perfect. In fact a lot of what I tried to do was not perfect. I had learned very brutally on imposing standards around laundry management. However, what I inherited from my mum was the need to get things done regardless of how I felt but getting things done on my long list of things was a way, like my mum, I coped with stress and the responsibilities life placed on me. I had an almost robotic approach to study because I did not put enough effort into 'how' I expressed what I knew but felt that memorizing everything in long lists was a way in which I could excel regardless of the form that knowledge took on paper. There was no reflection or critical thought about what I was being taught. My approach to education was derived from books as my father had taught me but to me books were just receptacles of facts. I underestimated the extent to which so called knowledge was contested. Because my politics were slightly left of centre and my lecturers were of a similar disposition it was enough to agree at face value with their interpretation of economic ideas.

Our main economic test for the first year was a book called Begg, Dornebush and Fistcher or as Mr. Harrison called it – Beg, Borrow and Steal it from your Mates. This was a huge six-hundred page book but was one of about seven basic texts with reading lists for each term and each of the three subjects that I did. This meant in my first year that there was an autumn and spring reading list for Politics, Economic and Social History and Economics. It was impossible to read everything that the lecturers required us to. To write a couple of 3,000 word essays required ideally reading eight or nine books in the space of a month with a couple of weeks left to write up. This was impossible at first and I had to read a booklet on speed reading. In the booklet you were told how to 'gut' a book in a nights reading. Speed reading involved sucking up information from the text with the speed of the reading determined by how quickly your eyes moved across the page. I found that the essence of the topics a book covered could be ascertained from its introduction. This meant that on some occasions there may only be a need to read one or two relevant chapters. Furthermore, reading the conclusion to a book was often the best way of getting its essence if you were short of time. Speed reading involved reading the first and last sentences of paragraphs more slowly because the essence of the topic was likely to be focused on here. Furthermore, when 'attacking' a book you had to have the essay question in your mind so that you only sucked in relevant information and were therefore 'skim reading' with a purpose in mind.

Against the main books we were required to read were Bernard Crick's 'In Defence of Politics', which was an introduction to political theory, 'Politics in the USA' by Vile an introduction to American Politics, David S. Lands 'The Unbound Prometheus' the story of European Industrialization in the Nineteenth Century, a book by Glass on the application of mathematics to Economic problems and a book by Peter Matthias called 'First Industrial Nation' – an account of

Britain's Industrialization. These were basic books I read, I never really ventured much into the reading lists because I struggled to speed read, relying heavily on my lecture notes for assistance in the structuring of my essays.

In the early 1980's word processing was a new phenomenon only used by people who could afford what were then expensive word processors. Essays therefore had to be written by hand. Quite often this meant that despite writing a first draft in which I often cut and pasted in the old fashioned way (with scissors and Sellotape) and I ended up having to use a great deal of Tippex in the final editing phase. One of our economic history tutors, Mr. Clarke commenting on my excessive use of Tippex on one essay suggested I bring a tin of white Dulux paint and a brush to the exam with me.

I struggled with the sheer volume of work required and the competing demand of socializing to combat any potential feelings of loneliness. Being away from home, particularly living with Duncan meant I lived in a relatively noise free environment and had a condition conducive to concentration. However, in practice I relied very heavily on my lecture notes and was only able to refer and read about three to four books per essay.

I spent most of my first year worrying about passing my exams. I felt that college had been a very poor academic preparation. I felt like a fraud, as if I were not as bright as everyone else and the exam period would be the time when I was found out. I struggled to write clear English Grammar in my politics essays and failed my first essay. Mortified, I read a book recommended to me on reading skills. I passed my politics exam by the skin of my teeth. I was a borderline candidate and they had a meeting about me. They decided I could proceed to my second year because I had attended all my political tutorials (very unusual for most students) and because my assessed essays had shown a steady improvement throughout the year. I just scraped home in Economics as well which meant I decided to combine Economic History with Economics so that I could work towards my strengths. This meant instead of working for an Economics degree I was now doing a Joint Honours.

It would be difficult to get through an account of my undergraduate years without a colorful look at some of the lecturers.

Mr. Skinner was, like most of the department, left of centre on the political spectrum. One day he thought he would try to shoot down Mrs. Thatcher's Monetarist approach to Economic Management. I had grasped at college, by reading Victor Keegan's notebook in *The Guardian,* that Mrs. Thatcher was trying to control inflation by controlling the supply of money. However, the governments name for its Monetarist approach was called the Medium Term Strategy or

MTFS as it was often abbreviated in the broadsheets. The lecturer said that Mrs. Thatcher's understanding of Economics could be understood by her upbringing, being brought up by a father who owned a grocery shop. He then continued in his sexist analysis. Her approach therefore was that the country could not spend more than it got in revenue from taxes, even temporarily. This fitted in with the idea, so he said of Mrs. Thatcher's experience as a housewife who could not overspend on her weekly shopping budget. The idea of the balanced budget so discredited after the Great Depression of the 1930's had now come back into fashion. Because Mrs. Thatcher's understanding of Economic management was so disparaged by Leicester academics they referred to it, so he said, as MTFS – MRS THATCHER'S FATHER'S SHOP.

Our Economic History tutor was Derek Aldcroft, subject of many homophobic jibes from students (behind his back). He was a Thatcherite and referred to three-million unemployed as a mere delayed consequence of over manning in British manufacturing in the 1950's and 1960's. He admitted however that inflation had been conquered in the 1980's not by the government's failure to control the money supply but deteriorating terms of trade with what we then called Third World countries. In other words, inflation was conquered by making people in developing countries poorer.

Our math's tutor was a fascinating man. Mr. Gibson was the closest I have ever come across to a man who could make anything mathematical interesting. He admitted to students he drooled over pictures of Harley Davidson bikes. This made me ask a question – was Mr. Gibson a 'born again' biker or was he a guy going through amid-life crisis? None of the stuff he taught was that difficult, merely 'O' Level math's applied to Economic problems. He did make us laugh when he plotted the number of trees on one axis and the number of dogs' pees on the other. The graph got referred to as the trees and the pees. This reminded me of something our Politics lecturer Mr. Maynor said. He said the weather is so dry in Arkansas that the trees followed the dogs around.

Then there was the great Economic History lecturer Mr. Fearon. He lectured about American Economic History like it was a bedtime story. He did not present the controversies, the arguments or debates, merely the story. You could even picture the scenery for yourself in the 1870's in the mid west plains of the United States on the 'Chisholm Trail' as he gave a lecture on American agriculture in the late 19th Century. He described to us the scene of Britain in the 1930's and surprisingly told us if you were lucky enough to have a job then you were not only comparatively well off but experienced a vast improvement in your living standards during this period. I got the feeling he did not like Edgar J. Hoover and was more a fan of FD. Roosevelt's 1930's New Deal (sounds vaguely New Labour to me).

The most effective way Mr. Fearon made himself a comedian in lectures with his vast knowledge of President, Lyndon Baines Johnson quotes. The funniest was when President Johnson was talking to his Canadian Economic advisor J.K. Galbraith. President Johnson, explained to his advisor why he did not like economic jargon. He said 'To me when people speak economic jargon it's a bit like pissing down the inside of your trouser legs, it might give you a nice sensation but it's not nice for the people standing around'. Apparently, President Johnson (LBJ) was renowned for dictating to his secretary even from a toilet cubical. Once it was said that Richard Nixon called Robert Kennedy a Carpetbagger for standing for election outside his home state. LBJ said that basically Richard Nixon didn't know what a Carpetbagger was and he said if he did then he'd be one. LBJ also said 'I wouldn't call President Ford dumb but I don't think he has the capacity to chew gum and walk in a straight line at the same time'.

The biggest joke in the politics department was the fact that Mr. Maynor, a lecturer from the US was in fact a specialist in Indian Politics. He was due to lecture us on American politics one day when he appeared in the lecture hall suddenly very late and very hassled. He explained that because the Indian President Mrs. Ghandi had been shot he was going to be inundated with requests for television and radio interviews.

My favorite lecturer though was Professor Pete Jackson. He blamed the recession of the early 1980's on the government's policy of maintaining a high exchange rate by ensuring that the real levels of interest rates were kept artificially high. He said the real levels of interest rates were determined by the actual level of interest rates relative to the rate of inflation. The actual level of interest rates seemed historically low but exceeded the level of inflation to a large extent meaning the cost of borrowing was suicidially high to businesses. Jacking up (his term) the level of interest rates, including the minimum lending rate during the initial period of high inflation in 1980 had thrown people unnecessarily out of work and had destroyed the manufacturing base in this country. Professor Jackson was particularly scornful of economists at Liverpool University especially an Economist who favored the government called Professor Patrick Minford. The theory of Economics espoused by Patrick Mitford was called the Theory of Rational Expectations. The essential idea behind the theory was that any government intervention in the economy would be read by consumers and businesses who would be able to understand the effect of such policies and behave as economic agents in a way to neutralize the effects of any government economic policy. The theory went that the neutralization effect was going on all day even when people got up to watch the morning news. Professor Jackson said – I'm not sure how you feel at 7am in the morning but even as an Economist myself I am not thinking about government Economic policy when I am eating my Cornflakes first thing in the morning.

My favorite lecture was given by Phil Fearon describing the crisis of capitalism in the United States in the early 1930's. Sometimes markets were not able to connect supply and demand he said. He painted a picture of unemployed people in the big American cities starving because they had no money for food with the simultaneous picture of a glut of produce rotting in rural areas because there was no financial demand for what had been grown. He argued that only government intervention would prevent falling prices, wages and employment would reverse the economic madness.

There was one lecturer Dr. Harrison who seems over keen to appear trendy to students. He felt his expertise in the Economics of Tax evasion was a real wease but what offended me more was his attempt to come out with any old joke to please students even if these jokes had racist or stereotypical overtones.

The quality of my assessed work improved with time from a first year when I handed in some very dire efforts. I remember quite clearly handing in a piece of work depicting a demand and supply curve for a commodity where it was obvious I did not understand income and substitution effects. The lines on the diagram depicted were all colours of the rainbow in what Mr. Bradbury described as 'very psychedelic'. I also mixed up the wartime coalition minister Ernest Bevin with the founder of the NHS Aneurin Bevan in my first politics essay for which I attained 39%.

In my final year I excelled at Macro-Economics (the economics of a whole country). We were being taught cutting edge theories on Economic management by Professor Peter Jackson who was clearly a fan of Professor Layard (who was dubbed a neo-Keynesian). Layard believed in the immediate post war interventionist economics but that intervention needed to take account of some economic aspects of the then Thatcher government and it's pre-occupation with the money supply. In this topic I was getting essays back that average 72-73%.

My final substantial piece of work was a 10,000 word dissertation on Development Economics in Third World Countries. The exact question was to identify what made foreign aid effective in terms of economic growth in countries with different types of economies. I was surprised that this topic was not more popular with students at large because of the recent publicity around the Live Aid concert. The statistical (or empirical) analysis involved measuring the relationship between foreign aid and economic growth in six countries which involved tediously pouring over World Bank

Reports and making hundreds of manual calculations. I was to end up with a high mark for my efforts. My supervisor for the topic was a man from India called Subrata Ghatak. He was extremely effective in communicating what was required and I only needed to meet him three times to complete the project.

My period as an undergraduate was, more than any other period of my life, when I explored my own identity in relation to other people my age. The problem was that I was a bit serious and did not identify with what I regarded as the frivolous antics of my contemporaries. However, the most influential person in changing my outlook was a fellow student from Huddersfield called Sean Lewis. I met Sean in my second year when he was my neighbour in Mary Gee student residences. From day one I was to get an ear bashing of the Duran Duran single "Planet Earth" on repeat when I was trying to study. I vented extreme anger at Sean and eventually things toned down a bit.

From the age of ten to nineteen I had lived my life out of a book but now I was bombarded with the need to read so much and for so long that I needed similar stimulation but in a way where I could put my brain into neutral. Furthermore, this need for stimulation needed to be part of my craving for collecting things.

Then one day I decided to build an album collection which would not conform to what was regarded as the decadent sounds of the 1980's but which I could build myself without reverence to the most popular radio stations. I was a bit poncey believing that once I developed a taste for Beethoven this music was necessarily more refined and sophisticated than the musical tastes of my contemporaries (that's why I collect eighties compilation albums presently).

Most importantly, Beethoven was something I could put on if Sean decided to play Duran Duran, after all it's better being distracted by your own noise than anyone else's. Sean turned out to be very good natured about our rivalry and eventually I looked up to him. He made light hearted comments about my lack of fashion sense and because I wore flares and patterned pullovers he called me "Reindeer man". I then got some fashion advice from him and spent money on clothes which shocked my mum.

In the autumn of 1985 I was really enjoying to get to know my flat mates at Mary Gee student residences. The kitchen, at Mary Gee which I shared with Sean and a couple of other flat mates must have been a breeding laboratory for a new strain of Salmonella. All I knew was that on the geography field trip to Spain Sean and some of his flat mates were the only people not to go down with food poisoning. Our kitchen must have been an excellent inoculation for them.

Another person I got to know very well in our block was Youen Effendi an Overseas (I think from Malaysia) student. He put us all to shame with his ability to stir fry food and to concoct weird and wonderful cocktails. He found like many people, my sense of humour based on obscure puns either predictable or just plain silly. I learned a great deal about fashion as he was a snappy dresser and knew how to make women feel comfortable around him. Youen and Sean were regulars on the nightclub scene until their overdrafts became a problem.

Jerry, another Mary Gee inmate together with his friend Guy hosted many parties. The arrival of guests was normally preceded by a couple of hours of painstaking arrangements which included the selection of the right wine.

I heard a strange noise across the landing one night. It sounded like Beethoven's 5th Symphony except it was not coming from my room. On further investigation it came from Guy's room, normally a refuge for heavy rock music (so out of fashion in the 1980's). Guy came to the door and openly admitted that I had converted him to Beethoven. What a coup. I couldn't wait to tell Sean.

It did not take long for some of our flat mates to set up the flat as a regular venue for War Games meetings. They tended to rearrange all the tables and put hundreds of soldiers on them in an attempt to re-enact various battles of historical significance. An exception to this was Thursday evening which everyone knew was Star Trek night.

I had (until meeting Sean) always been sure of who I was and what my purpose in life was all about. However, I started a process of constantly comparing myself to my contemporaries after January 1986 when I met someone whom I regarded as special. Rejection from this person was to cause my first identity crisis. Then I began constantly asking myself whether I was normal. Basic decisions even around the selection of an album or what to wear became agonizing as I analysed obsessively how those decisions appeared to fellow students. In my world everything I did had an impact on how others perceived me. Suddenly I didn't want to be different any more. Suddenly I wanted to fit in with my peers. This was the start of the first student crisis period.

CHAPTER TWO

THE INEXPLICABLE EXPERIENCE THAT BECAME LABELLED AS SCHIZOPHRENIA

When you experience what you perceive as love from a woman for the first time, it turns your world upside down. At the age of twenty I had not felt that I had been loved by my mother even though she had told me I was loved. Love up until then had been a couple of schoolboy crushes but nothing that was reciprocated.

It seems on January 6th 1986 that I had encountered reciprocal love from a woman. In reality all it was, was Janet (name anonymised) who had initiated a conversation, smiled at me and asked a few nosey questions. The whole process of this misunderstanding was experienced by me as rejection. It resulted in a nagging emotional pain that took me ten years to get over.

Janet was a short, petite, freckled woman with long hair cut to a fringe who always wore a pink felt coat. She could smile in a way that could light up her deliriously engaging eyes. It seems from her interaction with others that she was a very popular woman.

After a very warm initial conversation I was mystified by the attention from her but dismissed it as a one-off. However, about a week later our eyes met from a short distance as I ascended the basement stairs of the Attenborough Lecture Theatre. Again she gave me an engaging smile. This was the crucial point at which I perceived that she felt something towards me. It did not occur to me that she might have a partner or even that a great deal more evidence was needed before I committed my feelings. However, I did commit myself and fell headlong in love in that momentary glance.

At the time I had not realized that I had over the course of my childhood and adolescence become a very obsessive person. Not only was I obsessive but to some extent I had a huge need to feel in control and had never had to deal with a great deal of uncertainty. I had never been in a relationship with a woman that I could even call a close friend. Much of my life was about reaching academic goals within the framework of a tight rigid routine. Such coping strategies had been learned from my foster mother and to be quite honest I did not know any other way to manage.

With my feelings committed to Janet I planned to literally go and talk to her when our paths next crossed and to impose myself through a lengthy conversation aimed at getting to know her better.

The opportunity to talk to her materialized a few days later as she left the Student Union Shop. The conversation started okay and I found she lived at College Hall. She then asked me a question the significance of which I did not realize until about 18 months later. She asked me whether I knew anyone from Leicester University Rugby team. I do not remember any more of the conversation except that I did most of the talking. On reflection I feel I mad the mistake of not asking whether she had a partner and towards the end of our conversation, throwing caution to the wind, I suggested the opportunity that we could go out together in the future.

I was to find out that Janet was good at keeping calm in our encounters and taking her at face value she seemed amenable to my suggestion. However, she may not have been able to express herself at that meeting. She may well have had to think about how she would handle me when we next met.

I remember looking forward with great relish to meeting Janet as she left the next Macro-Economics lecture. However, as I approached her outside the lecture hall she defied my attempts to talk to her by hiding her face and running towards Percy Gee Students Union Building. I stood momentarily feeling humiliated not knowing what to do next. After a pause I entered the Percy Gee building looking for Janet. I found her sitting next to friends in the Student Union bar burying her face into someone's lap as I stared at her in the distance one of her friends came to me and explained that she had entertained thoughts of a friendship with me but had changed her mind and would continue to pursue her relationship with her boyfriend.

I was still in a state of shock. However, I did completely believe in the story offered by Janet's friend. I could believe that she did not have the courage to explain to me that she was already in a relationship. I felt that she had purposely humiliated me. Reflecting on it twenty years later I feel that I had really backed Janet into a corner. People can behave in pretty extreme ways when they feel cornered.

I was to find over the next few years that whilst obsession is a key quality in setting and achieving life time goals, it can damage and even wreck relationships. I also found that my yearning to rebuild the non existing relationship with Janet and my inability to accept rejection were to lead me on a journey that would push my life to devastation by the end of June 1987.

I kept the bedrock of my routine around study, running and social activity together but at the back of my mind I was deeply hurt and refusing to acknowledge feelings of emptiness. However, I did not acknowledge let alone confront these feelings. I chose instead to pursue a distraction coping strategy telling myself instead that there wasn't a problem at all. The consequence of this was that the pressure built up over the next 18 months to a point where I psychologically imploded.

From correspondence with Janet's tutor, nearly ten years later, I was to find that Janet and other students regarded me as a loner and a misfit. When I found this out I was a bit hurt to say the least. I certainly did not feel the need to conform to peer pressure but to describe me with such unpleasant labels is a sign that many communities cannot deal with, let alone accept difference.

I resolved after my humiliation that I would ignore Janet if our paths crossed again. However, when I did meet her in Queen's Hall one lunchtime, she talked to me and I found myself responding after a moment's pause that signified indecision. The incident led to unresolved feelings. Over the next months I was to give some contradictory signals.

For example, in the middle of January I bought a Valentine's card for Janet and gave it to her after a lecture, not knowing that Valentine's Day was not until February. I wrote all the positive adjectives I could think of and put them into this card which she accepted without saying much.

On another occasion I ignored Janet as she walked past me in the snow. Then I felt an agonizing sense of guilt afterwards. In the weeks immediately after my rejection I went into the student bar on about a dozen occasions during lunchtime. I felt bad about this because I never thought you could relax like this during your lunch break. I mourned the lack of socializing that I had had with my peer group. I stopped and played with the pinball machines fifty yards from where Janet was sitting but felt powerless to go and talk to her.

I also went to what was then called the 'Mega-disco' on Friday's hoping to bump into Janet or perhaps getting to know someone else. Quite often I went on my own but sometimes I was able to persuade Dave Jackson and Gerald Bane to go. I used to dance in an extremely energetic way hoping that I would attract the attention of other women on the dance floor. On reflection it probably put people off and reinforced my reputation as someone who was anything but normal.

Without realizing it, I was beginning to embark on a process of continual self analysis. I defined myself as someone who had been different from my peers and suddenly there was urgency about the need to fit in.

My feelings about the need to conform affected every part of my life. I dressed like other students, got a regular haircut and tried to change my image. Part of this transformation was about getting trendy music and again I sought advice from Sean. Suggestions for music included the Cocteau Twins, U2 and Joy Division. My neighbour even persuaded me to venture into 20th Century classical music. Sean also suggested that I watch the Tube presented by Jools Holland and Paula Yates.

I felt that the student community at Leicester University was very small and close-knit. I perceived that a change in my image from clothing to music would get back to Janet and force her to re-evaluate me. I realized that a close relationship was impossible but it was something that I dreamed about every day. I hoped in the very least that we could be friends. Again from correspondence with Janet's tutor I learned that there may have been a perception from Janet that she was being pursued. I did however put strict limits around the way I behaved, limits that were to remain in place until I psychologically imploded at the end of June a year later. I could have found out where Janet lived from her friends but refrained from asking. I could have also found out her whereabouts after lectures but again I refrained from doing this. The only strategy I had was to go about my everyday business in the hope that the news of my transformation of my image would get back to Janet.

In the spring of 1987 I was at a psychological and emotional peak In the Macro-Economics module entitled 'Growth, Instability and Uncertainty' I was receiving back essays with marks of over 70%. In middle distance races I had nearly beaten every other member of the Leicester University Cross Country / Athletics Team. I won a couple of races even on the track. However, over the coming weeks the wheels would slowly come off.

In my final year I not only had to get through my final exams, I also had to get a job. On reflection it would have been better to get through my final exams, have a break, then get a job. However, I piled on needless pressure on myself and what made things worse was that I did not reduce the quantity or quality of training as an athlete. An athlete who had tried to keep up with me had broken his hip.

Another pressure I had was the difficulty of going back to live with my parents after living for the best part of three years in relative independence. I understood that going back to them would mean restrictions on my lifestyle. The journey back to Birmingham would also mean not ever being able to meet Janet again. But the point of no return had been reached with Janet 18- months previously. Acknowledging the prospect of making no future progress with Janet made me extremely angry. It came to a head a couple of months before graduation. One night after going to a student gig I decided to express how I felt in writing. I began in a conciliatory tone but it was not long before the anger blurted out across the page as each crossing out led me to express myself more directly. I stormed down to College Hall armed with a letter expressing my anger at her. I knocked randomly on a downstairs room and the person who answered happened to know her and said she was on a skiing holiday. I then angrily put the letter in his hand and demand he give it to her on her return.

LIVING OUT OF THE BOOK

I had noticed from the way some people talked to me that they had had conversations with others in which they discussed my welfare. For example a woman I had vaguely known from Villiers Hall started to talk to me in an animated way. She was an attractive woman and I had misread the initial clues and felt she was chatting me up. However, she asked if she could talk with me in the library. It was about 9am. and her style of conversation changed when in the library to questions about how I was feeling, was I worried about anything and as I answered each question she seemed to be ticking off her mental checklist, 'Erm…. That's normal' after about ten minutes of this she abruptly ended the conversation, probably on her way to a lecture.

I also happened to visit my old hall Mary Gee residences and bumped into Sean who talked to me briefly about my improved taste in music (he mistook a Paul Young cover version of 'love will Tear us Apart' for Joy Division). He also agreed it was extremely funny that I had compared one of his tall flat mates to 'Lurch' from 'The Adam's family'. He said he had talked about me to his mate (a mutual acquaintance from our first year at Villiers) and we both agreed how good the Joshua tree album was. Sean even said that he had tried my techniques of essay writing to great effect.

It was quite clear that even my efforts to conform were deviations from the norm and creating conversation amongst other students.

It is an extremely dangerous habit to imagine what other people are thinking without substantial effort to back it up with evidence. Such habits can cause insomnia in the very least.

Just before my finals I had a night when I could not sleep. I felt claustrophobic in this close-knit student community. My strategy of image change and trying to appeal to Janet through the grapevine was not working. Because it was not working I imagined the worst and felt that rather than it seducing Janet it was making her antagonistic, irritated and turning her against me. The process of hearing voices is a very subtle one. First I felt that my image change was not working then I felt that this may be because Janet and her friends were against me. This seemed to be borne out by a number of unfortunate situations where various people who had been casual acquaintances from College Hall shouted things at me like 'lovers tiff' and insinuating that they felt they had been used.

Once you start to feel people are against you, the next stage to hearing voices is that you start to feel people are against you. Then you start to imagine what they might be thinking. The next stage is that you feel you know what people are thinking and before long everyone is against you and you feel you have a unique gift of psychological telepathy. When you hear positive voices no one notices. I had felt Janet was warming towards me in the summer of 1986. The reason for this was that I had run in a sponsored race called 'Run the World'. I had noticed that Janet had been a spectator at this event. I had finished in the top six of this race. The next day when I was completing my exam she finished her exam earlier and walked the long way out of the exam and brushed past my table. Some of her college Hall mates had honked their horn in a friendly manner to me after the screening of 'Amadeus' at the Student's Union Building. Positive voices do not interfere or make you anxious. However, negative voices do and before long the speed of your thinking increases more and more as your paranoia increases. Because I could not handle the increasing volume of voices and quantity of people persecuting me co-ordination is lost between the thoughts which means you lose logic between one thought and another as your thinking darts about. Listening to someone with a mental health issue in the mist of psychosis can sometimes mean that you hear them jump from one topic to another with no apparent connection between them.

My feelings of anger and frustration at Janet had been building up since Easter 1987. Shortly after coming back I had an evening when I could not get to sleep. The focus of my frustration was that I felt Janet was talking negatively about me to her friends but as these perceptions of Janet's conversation became more intense I felt that she had for some reason been talking to my athletics club mates back in Birmingham. By the time the voices had reached this stage I was walking to Elm Road Houses to Victoria Park. Half-way down Knighton Road I broke into a crying fit. However, by the time I reached the War Memorial in the park I had completely regained my exposure. I realized I had been psychotic and I had a clear choice. I could either go to my tutors and be exempted from my exams or try to get through the pressure of my finals after which I felt everything would be okay. I opted for the latter.

On a final visit home before my exams I was still in negative self analysis mode, thinking myself to be of a low mental age. My foster parents gave me the reassurance I needed but this was only a brief lull in the process of pulling myself apart.

Another student had told me of the drug induced student who had 'tripped out' in the exam room and written a three-hour exam paper by failing to move his ball point from the one line he had written on. He had therefore written 2,000 words on a single line by continuously writing over what he had written.

My exam performance was mediocre and I had a habit of indecision which meant I never completed a single exam paper and had presentation that was marred by crossings out. After my final paper on June 4th 1987 I stumbled into a bar after completing my final exam.

I phoned my foster parents just after my exams stating that I would not return home. I had convinced them I found accommodation in Leicester but I had nowhere to stay and was merely trying to delay the inevitable.

About three weeks after my final exams I went to the Attenborough building to collect my results. In those days they displayed everyone's class of degree on the board. I looked amongst the Economics and Economic History listings for my results and found that I had attained a second class degree lower division or a 2:2. I glanced across to the Economics results and found that Lloyd Gutteridge had got a First (over 70%). Then my eyes descended down the list to Janet who had got a 2:2, the same as me. I was not disappointed but I knew it would be more difficult to get a job without a 2:1 degree. A second class degree higher division would have signified that I had attained between 60-70% in my overall result. I was pleased I had got through but I had an empty feeling inside that my yearning to keep in contact with Janet would be unfulfilled. The emptiness was a feeling I had because I was finally coming to terms with loss in my life. For the first time in my life I was actually grieving. I had experienced failure in my life but never losing someone special. What's more, I was powerless and I did not know how to cope with such an overwhelming sense of loss.

What made things worse was that my insight into what had actually been going on in this close-knit student community started to make itself apparent.

I found out a number of things that that caused me to think very negatively towards Janet and her friends in the weeks after my exam. Firstly I had thought that, though my music was loud from my flat, I had a reasonable sense of taste. However, after the day after the landslide election in 1987 I had put a slogan on my window 'Divide and Rule'. When I went next door I heard a couple of the students making negative comments about this sticker. When I saw them they were perfectly nice to my face but in another meeting with them they told me more disturbing things. They described a small woman who kept visiting and always insisted on watching skiing. Knowing how Janet liked skiing it was not too far fetched to me that she and my neighbours had been spying on me. Another visitor to their block may have been her partner whom I had seen in various poses of PDA (public displays of affection) with Janet. He was described as a blonde rugby player built like a big brick shit house. Furthermore, a neighbour drew a big face on his window with tears on it. I did not know whether these things were a coincidence, and whether to ignore these issues but in the end I went next door and confronted everyone. I left in tears despite their reassurances that they were not against me.

It was about a week after finding out the results of my finals that I became irreversibly ill. I started to feel that Janet was in touch with everyone I knew and knew everything about me. I tried to confront the voice of Janet hoping it would stop tormenting me but it went on and on and on and on. Janet was alternating between sexually provocative behaviour and criticism directed towards me. She kept throwing me on and off the scent in sexually provocative behaviour that was trying to provoke a response. It got to a point where I could no longer cope with the number of voices and their intensity and their ferocity. The only way I could get rid of the voices was to confront their focal point and that meant tracking down Janet.

However, I could not do this because she started to turn on the charm. She started to be very warm to me. So warm that after a while I started to feel that I could propose marriage. At this point my critical self analysis crept in as I could not imagine being good enough to marry her. I then reflected on my absent minded nature and the fact that even if I fulfilled my boyhood dream of becoming a naval officer it would not be good enough for her. I begged her to give me a chance, even just a foot in the door but no positive response came.

I was appealing one last time to this all powerful panel of voices hoping that if I could function in a high powered graduate job that this would be good enough for Janet.

I then tried to get rid of the voices by relaxing. I relaxed by reading the student newspaper 'Ripple'.

My mind was in such a state of overdrive that within minutes of picking up this newspaper, I found the stories in the magazine seemed to be written about me. Not only this, but the paper was written in a way that seemed well informed about my current state of mind. One minute I was reading an innocent story about Beaumont Hall Gardens, the next I felt there were subliminal messages which were directed at me about the Gardens being a venue for a suicide pact between two past students. The story was both a warning and potential prophesy to me.

After I put the paper down I summoned sufficient concentration to make myself some porridge. Whilst waiting for the contents of the saucepan to cook I felt I was psychologically in touch with a panel of people who were deciding about my future with Janet. I kept pleading with this panel. I admitted to them that I was absent minded and a bit of a scatter brain and that in some ways I was not good enough for Janet but I promised and pleaded about being better in future. I even promised to shape up and join the Royal Navy so that I could one day be good enough for her.

I had been able to cook the contents of the saucepan well. I then poured the contents of the saucepan in a bowl. However, my concentration drifted again as I began to ape the behaviour of a small child scooping up spoonfuls of porridge and dropping it back into the bowl repeatedly. While I was engaged in this activity one of my flat mates walked in with his partner. They stared at me briefly with tears in their eyes, my flat mate having to hug and console his partner momentarily before they left quietly.

After leaving my breakfast half-eaten I became distracted. I could hear Janet's voice. At times it seemed it was teasing me. The only thing was I could seem to relieve the mental agony was to confront the voice directly. That meant tracking down Janet. It was about 6am as I decided to go where I thought she lived, which was college Hall.

As I headed up Elms Road on route to College Hall I had a brief moment of insight. It seemed to me that I was experiencing the world in a very strange way. I felt that the odd person I could see might be a spy. The road sighs seemed to prophesy something. The next moment I was challenging this idea in my head.

When I arrived at my destination I headed towards 'A' block where I thought Janet might be. I did not know her address so I reckoned that if I knocked on every door I would eventually encounter her. I started to knock on each door with no responses from most and as this continued to happen I became more upset and hysterical. After a short time I realized that my quest was futile. I then knelt on the floor banging my fists on the ground in a massive crying fit. I began to plan how I was going to throw myself under the nearest car or bus.

Within moments I could hear someone calling from the stairs. I walked to the stairs and encountered a bearded, middle-aged man whom I was to find out was the college warden. He quietly asked me if I was okay. Then he asked whether I needed any help. I told him I just could not go on.

He took me downstairs. I expected to be told off but he seemed very friendly in a quiet sort of way. When we got downstairs he headed towards his living quarters. He introduced me to his wife and in the background his children were getting ready for school. I immediately unloaded my troubles onto this man but he did not seem shocked he merely told me how Janet had lived there the year before and had gone to live in a privately rented house. After a while he said that my colours had returned. He was very friendly and somehow I felt glad he so understood.

He then told me that on the way to taking his children to school he would drop me off at the Student Health Centre.

Upon arrival at the centre I lost the moments of clarity that I had had with the College Hall warden as my mind began to shoot of in all sorts of tangents. For example, whilst I was sitting opposite a nurse who was eating, I resorted back to the babyish behaviour that I had exhibited earlier. I was consuming food off the nurse's plate with my fingers. In the background the news programme on the radio seemed to be churning out current affairs issues that had subliminal messages based on observations of my behaviour.

It was not long before I was interviewed by the Student Health Centre doctor. When I asked him if I was mad he patronized me by saying 'I suppose we're all mad'. He interviewed me at length and as he did so I lost my brief moment of insight and began admitting everything that was rushing into my head.

I began reflecting on a question about current affairs and thinking about current issues in *The Guardian*. I then began to feel that my interpretation of what was in the news was not only important and unique but a form of prophesy. I then began to believe I was a prophet. Within seconds of this I felt I predicted an apocalypse and this was tied in with the Biblical chapter of Revelation. I had never read 'Revelation', knew nothing about what it said but this did not stop me having grandiose delusions about feeling that I could be the second coming of Christ.

I was then left in a room on my own. My eyes focused about me. I was surrounded by first aid dummies. I began to feel like an alien. Perhaps I did not belong to the world of ordinary human beings. I felt dehumanized and that like these dummies I needed to undergo a ritual to become fully human. If I became fully human perhaps Janet might be able to love me.

I then boarded the ambulance which I felt was a bit melodramatic for someone with my issues. On the way to the hospital I had more interaction with the voices that were supposedly deciding my future with Janet.

I arrived at the hospital engaged in a major crying fit. Upon arrival at Leicester General Hospital I started to wreak all sorts of havoc. Not long I got through the door, I was asked by an elderly woman what my name was. I stuttered in response to this question being undecided between my birth name Matthew and my adopted name Philip. I had my leg pulled about that through the rest of my seven week stay.

I walked towards the patients lounge to watch a history programme narrated by the BBC Mastermind winner Fred Housego. I could not hear what he was saying but I began to feel he was describing the fortifications of a castle with a deep underground system of tunnels and listening posts that was somehow listening in on me. This thought disturbed me and I began to swap channels in what was a captive audience. I finally settled for BBC2s coverage of Wimbledon.

This program seemed intriguing. It featured a match between the ageing and legendary Jimmy Connor's and the young Czech upstart Penfors. Everything I was sure of in my psychotic world was allied with Connor's whilst Penfors seemed allied to the psychotic forces that were unsettling me. Connor's was down two sets and 4-2 in the third set. Every point Penfors won seemed to cause me psychological pain whereas when Connor's won a point it lifted my spirits. I was interrupted in mid-match by the nurse who switched back to the original channel, much to the relief of the other patients.

I was then interviewed by a middle aged woman who claimed she was a social worker. She referred me to thoughts I had expressed earlier. I had felt that my psychological pain was the transfer of psychic energy from my natural mother because she had died. She claimed she had phoned round and informed me that my natural mother was still alive.

After the interview with the social worker I became suddenly very tired indeed. Then I remembered I had taken some medication soon after my arrival at the hospital. Within minutes I was shown to my bed where I slumped and immediately went to sleep.

There was a brief period of about three minutes when I awoke. In this window of opportunity I remembered what I had experienced the day before and became aware that I was now thinking perfectly rationally. I now allowed myself to think that I had been cured.

Then.... then, I stepped out of bed and realized the tablets they had given me as well as making me think straight had in fact slowed me down considerably. I walked only with a great deal of effort and it seemed to take every ounce of concentration that I had. I suddenly felt ten years older.

Walking was not the only activity that required an extreme effort. As I sat and read the paper I could only focus on one sentence at a time before momentarily dozing off.

I suddenly reflected on how disabled I had become and began to think about what this would mean. My disability placed doubt on whether I would ever get a job. It also placed a question mark over other lifetime milestones such as finding a lifelong partner and becoming financially independent enough to live away from my parents. It seemed that everything I had worked for at University was now in vain. I asked the nurses at medication time about my future but they gave me non committal responses.

In the end I decided to make the best of my situation and went about busily making friends on the ward. The woman who had pulled my leg over my name was a lady who had been admitted herself because the repossession of her house had caused her to have a breakdown. She was a calm person who seemed in good humour most of the time. It was difficult to see from her outward behaviour, which I regarded as normal, why she had been admitted in the first place.

However, there were a fair number of patients who caused me concern. For example, there was a young man called Steve. He was a small guy but what disturbed me was the powerful effect of medication on his overall demeanor. He looked completely sapped of energy and he moved round the ward with slow, laboured even robotic type movements. His face was almost mask-like and devoid of human expression. I asked myself weather I looked like this to other people.

There was a young woman, a law student on the ward who expressed her inner stress by drawing people with horrifyingly distorted faces. She had attempted to self harm a number of times. She told me she experienced depression most of the time.

I met one guy who was fond of traditional dancing and folk music. It was not long before I was told he had been admitted because his partner had been compulsively unfaithful to him.

I had a number of visitors during my stay. My first visitors were my foster parents. They smiled at me and struggled to open the conversation. They had been phoned by the ward when I was unwell and told that their son could barely remember his name. Naturally my parents were upset and my foster mother cried.

When they finally saw a psychiatrist they were told that I may have schizophrenia. It took another few months for me to be told of my suspected diagnosis. The psychiatrist was quite helpful and gave a laypersons description of the diagnosis. He said that when the brain became overactive the composition of the fluid connecting different parts of the brain changed. Normally the fluid in the brain pass signals from one part of the brain to the other. When the brain became overactive not only did messages get passed around but messages start to get made up in a process that would cause psychosis. This led to me believing things that had no relation to what was actually going on in the real world. The purpose of medication was to slow down the transmission of messages so that messages were not made up.

My first home leave with my foster parents was exciting, however I quickly became unwell because I started to feel this inner agitation and restlessness. Over the weekend this gradually became worse until I reached a point where I was in mental agony. I was to find out that such suffering was caused by the side effects of the medication. Within twenty minutes of arriving back on the ward I was given a tablet called Proclydine which enabled me to feel far more relaxed.

There was a period of time when my parents were exceptionally kind to me. They took me on excursions to Rutland Water and Newstead Abbey, but as the realization dawned on them that my recovery would take years rather than weeks the cracks soon showed in my foster mother's patience. My foster mother told me one day that I was not the Philip she once knew, 'you're a different Philip. We left the old Philip back in Leicester'. There was no apology for this and it was extremely upsetting to hear my foster mother talk this way. This was something I could not pull myself together from. Such frustration expressed by her merely made me feel even more negative about myself and my prospects. There seemed to be no hope.

Probably the most tense visit to me in hospital was by two of my university lecturers. They wore concerned expressions. They told me that my dissertation had been really good. Overall they lacked animation in their voices but seemed sad, calm and deadpan. I also received a visit from two of my student friends Dave and Gerard. They cheered me up no end because of their lively banter.

One day I put my running kit on an attempted to go for a run. It became obvious after a short jog that I could no longer produce enough adrenalin to run without slowing down after a short period of jogging to a point where I was once more resorting to a walking pace. My dream of becoming a top class athlete died that day. Again, much of what I had striven for in my life now seemed in vain.

During my stay I felt that therapy sessions aimed at improving my circulation were not age appropriate when I had previously considered a five mile steady run an easy session.

Then it was decided by ward staff that I would be well enough to attend the graduation ceremony after merely two weeks in hospital. I was excited. But when it came to the day trying on my gown on the ward made some patients think I was a headmaster or something.

There was a moment of panic when we all thought we were going to be late for the ceremony because my father could not seem to get out of a one way system en route to De Montefort Hall. When I arrived at campus there were clearly students who were surprised to see me.

In the Hall I clapped eyes on the College Hall warden who had helped me a couple of weeks before. He was part of the procession, he then saw me and winked. I saw Janet walk and collect her degree

And she seemed to avoid eye contact with everyone. I then received my degree with ritual applause.

I spotted Janet after the ceremony and went to talk to her. I asked her about her future plans and she told me she might stay on and do a Master's Degree. My foster mother was not happy with this. Earlier she told me there are plenty of fish in the sea. I could see she wanted me to move on but I felt unable to do that at the time. I also saw Gerard who collected his degree without a gown. He seemed in good spirits and in a similar mood to when he had visited me in hospital.

On the ward one day a woman asked me to go with her to the University. I asked the staff whether I could go and they asked whether I was attracted to her. After denying that I was we left for campus. We parted momentarily and I went to the Economics Department to track down someone who had been both my tutor and Janet's tutor at different times.

LIVING OUT OF THE BOOK

When I spoke to Dr. Catherine Price I explained I had had a nervous breakdown and asked whether Janet could be told of this. She agreed and then gave me a business card with both her work and home phone numbers on it. She said I should ring her if I needed any help or just keep in touch.

I then rejoined my friend and we went to a house in a posh suburb where an English lecturer lived. He too had had a nervous breakdown very much to do with his divorce. He showed us both down to his vast Aladdin's Cave of books. Then he asked me whether I liked classical music. I then said I liked Beethoven so we listened to the Ninth Symphony while we all sipped tea.

It was a very tragic situation. Rather than being an energetic, dynamic recent graduate I was instead a quiet, reserved, empty shell, a poor reflection of my former self. I was no longer articulate but had difficulty stringing sentences together. I had lost my drive and motivation and was largely indifferent and unemotional about everything around me. I had poor levels of mental energy, everything seemed a huge effort. The prospect of death seemed welcome – I dreamed of that eternal lie-in.

Over the next twelve months I was to be sacked as a volunteer at Elfrida Rathbone, prevented from finishing a placement at a local library and sacked as a clerical assistant at British telecom. I also found a job at a garage too stressful.

I saw my medication as an obstacle to achieving things. At outpatient appointments I argued that I was overmedicated and persuaded the psychiatrist to eventually reduce my dosage gradually until I came off medication completely. This was the only way I could see of escaping my diagnosis of schizophrenia and recovering my level of motivation both to work and to recommence my career as a middle distance runner. The risk of coming off medication became too much eventually and around 18-months after being admitted to Leicester General I would be a patient at Highcroft Hospital. I now accept that I am on medication for life and that society will thus, as it does, define me as a paranoid schizophrenic.

PART THREE.

MY RELAPSE.

I had suffered my first breakdown without knowing what had happened to me. It was not until a couple of months after leaving hospital that my Disablement Resettlement Officer, at the Job Centre, told me my diagnosis (she assumed I already knew it). My reaction upon realizing I was diagnosed with Paranoid Schizophrenia was one of relief, at least I had identifiable symptoms and my problems however difficult were now tangible. However, in the long term the implications of a lifelong dependency on medication (and the stigma associated with the schizophrenia label by the media and thus the general public) changed that view.

The perception of how I saw myself was drastically changed in the months after discharge from hospital. Most of the confidence I had spent my life building began to evaporate. The expectations of others towards me and of me towards myself lowered. My ambition therefore became limited. I had gone from wanting a high powered graduate job in July to be willing to accept any job by November. I was forced to stay in each night due to lack of money and the opportunity to earn some had vanished. Despite other peoples' perceptions of me changing, I still knew I had something to offer a potential employer and it was this self belief that kept me job hunting through periods of repeated rejections. People treat you differently when your status changes from promising undergraduate to mentally ill graduate. Suddenly people go from heaping praise and encouragement to wanting to shelter you from stress.

Whilst the psychiatric drugs I took controlled the illness they also (by the side effects) put up a barrier to people wanting or hoping to access the pre-illness persona. I still possessed latent ability but somehow the medication gave me that vegetated look preventing people from seeing that ability and preventing me from having the confidence to show them. Not surprisingly I equated lower doses of medication with the loosening of a mental straight jacket without realizing how I might try to overcompensate time lost when off the medication. Most people may think that someone who suffers a breakdown and a diminishing quality of life in the aftermath can be very emotional. It was true, I was depressed but not emotional. The medication put a brake on the emotions as well. Feelings of irritation, elation, attraction, anger and nervousness that many of us take for granted were dulled by 40mg of Flupenthixol Decoanate.

By coincidence or otherwise the timing of obtaining a job as a postal filling clerk (nearly 12 months on from the onset of my first illness) coincided with coming off psychiatric medication (injections). From this point on I felt I could put my illness behind me and turn over a new leaf.

By being preoccupied with holding down a job and re-establishing myself as a good club country/athletics runner (I was keen to make up for time lost) I neglected, as I had previously at University my life style.

In retrospect, I feel it was unwise that I added 50 miles a week training (some of which was very intensive) to what was a very physically demanding job. Furthermore, I rarely allowed myself the opportunity outside of sleep to sit down and unwind. When coming off my injections my doctor told me the risk period was 6-12months after coming off but it did not sink in that I might encounter 'cold turkey' so I went about my life inflicting different types of stress on myself as if invulnerable and cured.

I rarely cooked or ensured that I ate a regular or nutritionally balanced diet. So by running as much as I did, holding down a physically demanding job, not giving myself much chance to unwind and, only partially replenishing my reserves of energy (due to an inadequate diet) I was effectively running myself into the ground.
I had a warning of what was to come in October that year (1988) having to take two to three weeks off training resulting from burn out due to excessive training and racing. Despite allowing myself the opportunity to recharge my batteries, I threw myself back into the usual hectic routine. Around this time too I developed what I would

term to be an hyperactive, overbearing manner. The normal reserved persona had deserted me to be replaced by an eccentric nature. I became flippant and sarcastic, walking about with my foot in my mouth occasionally upsetting people. This was not an act to impress but very much a reaction to the pace of life I was leading. My speed of thought outpaced any inhibitions I had.

I feel there were two events that determined the eventual timing of my relapse. Namely, a visit to Leicester University and a cross country race too far. On the invitations of some of my Leicester University Cross Country Teammates I returned one weekend.

I did not for one moment anticipate the trauma this would cause me when I re-trod the footsteps of my first illness. Memories of my infatuation reached much closer to the surface of my conscious thoughts. All the nullifying effects of the drugs had become undone. It had been a while since I experienced emotional pain and like a tiny germinating seed my obsession for Janet returned.

Arriving back from my weekend to work (the University surroundings had very much reminded me of what I had attained) I became resentful of the illness I had suffered that had caused me to end up on a low paid, low status, dead end job. Over the coming weeks, despite an attempt to resist such thoughts, I started to feel it was Janet who had wrecked my career whilst still at the same time hoping for that chance in a million of meeting her, to seduce her.

LIVING OUT OF THE BOOK

One night I was so overwhelmed by anger and desire towards Janet that I was unable to sleep and in the early hours I embarked on the composition of a letter to my former Economics tutor. In this letter I condemned Janet's flirtatious behaviour describing what had happened between us, in the deluded hope that he had some ultimate sanction over Janet via his influence on the University Authorities. I suggested that we discuss my letter over dinner (for which I offered to pay) and that I would make a special visit to Leicester. Naïve though these assumptions were it helped calm me down and after posting the letter I was able to relax and soon went to sleep.

Leamington Spa had a cross country venue which was the toughest in the Midlands with its back breaking hill surrounded by a damp, extremely muddy course. It was a bit of a man killer to say the least. The race, the Senior Men's Warwickshire Cross Country Championships, involved running three circuits of this course. Half way round the first circuit I felt something inside me snap but no serious symptoms resulted and I soon forgot what had happened.

However, a week later when my brother got angry with my untidiness around the flat he screamed in anger at me so loud and for so long that the hollow feeling inside my chest that had happened during my last race, returned. The sensation was unpleasant and aggravated by the least physical effort. The condition only subsided when I was in a reclining position in peaceful surroundings. Paul must have felt he had an invalid for a brother. I knew instinctively that I was on the verge of a relapse and was able to, aided by a slightly improved condition, obtain Stelazine capsules which the doctor claimed would help me to become tired naturally. The tablets worked as intended but the course ran out a week before Christmas. I enjoyed the festive season and was able to relax fully for the first time since October.

However, before returning to work I attended an outpatient's appointment with my psychiatrist. I told her of the symptoms that I felt I had overcome. She responded by saying that I looked better that I had done in October and that many outpatient's suffered 'stress reactions' when withdrawing from medication. But nevertheless she felt it necessary to prescribe me some tablets to be taken if the so called 'stress reactions' reoccurred.

The symptoms re-emerged on the fourth day back at work and I had to leave the office at Midday in tears. I could not make the journey home in one burst, the symptoms seeming to debilitate me. I nevertheless made it home.

When I tried to review my prescription for Stelazine I was told that my medical records had been lost and that because of this I could not see the doctor. I explained the seriousness of the situation but the receptionists were adamant. Instead I was told to seek help by enlisting at a doctor's surgery with vacancies for new clients. Denied medication I was desperate. I began a futile journey across much of East Birmingham from surgery to surgery in need of help. After giving up this quest I visited Acocks Green Library on the way home and borrowed a book called "Self Help For Your Nerves" and sat on a park bench and read it religiously, ravenously digesting the section on insomnia and realizing the need to stay awake to return to a normal sleeping pattern. Unfortunately I fell asleep on the park bench for quite a while then returned home.

I lay in bed practising deep breathing exercises in line with the descriptions of a relaxation method outlined in my library book but the stage the illness had reached was too advanced for me to reverse what had happened. It was only when the audible delusions and accompanying symptoms of schizophrenia re-emerged in the next two days that I finally gave up my lone fight.

On Tuesday 8th January 1989 I awoke and my comprehension of what was going on bore no relation to reality. I felt that the cast of the Australian soap 'Neighbours' (when one of the cast used the term 'highly strung') were condemning my behaviour. I opened the door, I thought that a free calor gas canister had been delivered because some of my friends had talked on my behalf to the suppliers. Then I remembered that this very canister was the empty one I had left outside a couple of days before. Whilst I was aware I was ill it did not change my flawed perception of what was going on around me.

I went out for a run thinking that would help me relax but despite putting in intensive effort I slowed due to a lack of mental energy. I described this sensation to someone in a charity shop and they put it down to a milky drink I may have had. For a while I thought that someone had sneaked a sedative in my diet. Then, when I returned home, I remembered I had taken one of the pills that the psychiatrist had given me for 'stress reactions'. I was slipping into and out of reality like a yo-yo.

I developed a paranoia regarding the malfunctioning of some of the electronic equipment in the house and felt that one of my previous employment Training Officers, Fergus, had planted bugs around the whole flat so that most of the people who knew me could detect what I was thinking. I felt like a private detective in my quest to de-bug my flat. The interaction of the voices became so intense that on the next occasion I was thinking straight I realized I was in desperate need of hospital treatment. I boarded a bus but became restless and ended up walking the remaining two-miles to East Birmingham Hospital, breaking into crying fits at regular intervals.

Whilst talking to the security guard at the hospital, despite a valiant try, I was unable to keep my composure whilst describing my symptoms and ended up crying frantically. Fortunately, I was able to make myself understood. I was taken to an interview at the Yardley Green Unit with my psychiatrist who told the ambulance staff to put me on one of her wards at Highcroft Hospital.

On arrival at the hospital I was initially interviewed by a staff nurse in a nurse's station. I described people's negative feelings towards me and perceived he was blaming me as deserving such a lack or respect and started convulsing in yet another crying fit.

When I was subsequently interviewed by a ward psychiatrist I had completely recovered composure and explained everything to him in a dead pan manner.

Then I sat on a ward nest to a student nurse describing in a cynical authoritative way a "1984" (George Orwell novel) type scenario where a hidden authority outside of a democratic system was controlling and manipulating society with some sort of hidden agenda. I pointed top the ceiling referring to people in a hidden room upstairs making big decisions over our lives. I felt that some of my friends who had been in the Federation of Conservative Students had influence in the high ministerial ranks of government and that I could exert influence indirectly through them.

I also felt that for some reason I had suddenly become famous, that my destiny had always been to be famous and that the various personalities on TV had a message for me now I had come of age and my grooming for divine stardom had been completed.

Despite initial medication I needed PRN (extra medication) before I could gain what was my best nights sleep for weeks. The approach of the doctors to my illness was very different to my first breakdown at Leicester General. Then they heavily medicated me and my delusions vanished overnight. This time I would suffer more as my medication was gradually increased to its optimum dose which took two months. In that period (during which I experienced the partial, initial and temporary recovery from my illness) I was to suffer from some less tortuous delusions in varying degrees.

Early in the morning, on my first complete day on the ward, I asked for and was granted permission to visit the city centre. I had the misguided notion largely picked up from a distorted perception of a local news item from the TV that there was a reception committee to mark the incorporation of celebrity status. I walked down Livery Street to be blinded by a light reflected from a glass covered office tower. This ordinary sight seemed quite eerie to me.
Putting this block behind me I walked to Snow Hill House, the place where I thought the reception was waiting for me, slipped through the security on the staff entrance (without meaning to) and walked through every office until it dawned on me, on the 6th and top floor that this might be an ordinary council office on a routine day.
When walking past the entrance of the Central Library I was able to gain the right interpretation of

the local news item which I had seen on TV. It was a day to celebrate the 100th anniversary of the city's incorporation and Birmingham inhabitants were encouraged by the few library staff I could see walking about in Victorian clothes to go about in the contemporary costume of 1889.

On the bus trip back to the hospital ward I started to develop paranoia and imagined a "1984" (George Orwell novel) scenario with people everywhere I went observing my thoughts (spying) and trying to thwart my plans which I was formulating to detect them. For the first time in my life I felt that our "constitutional democracy" was just a façade behind which a small elite group of people were really in control of the country to such an extent that the actions of ordinary citizens were controlled. When I discussed my ideas with a few patients on the ward when I got back they fed my delusions by responding affirmatively to my new outlook on the world.

After a few days I started to carry a diary round with me everywhere I went documenting how I was feeling and putting on paper the thoughts that were going through my head.

One such feeling was a deluded realization that I had been contaminated by my University friends (?) with recreational drugs and that they had done this by 'spiking' my surroundings. An innocent junkie?

When watching "Crime watch UK" a feeling developed inside of me that I was a runaway criminal and that the programme was aimed at getting people to find me. I had a growing feeling I was guilty of some sort of abuse and that the reason I had forgotten my crimes was due to some form of amnesia that resulted from an abused childhood. These delusional thought "clouds" were not dwelling for long periods but were interspersed by rays of reality that shone through intermittently.

I seemed to be recuperating quite well when on a visit to pick up some items from my flat I heard the news of the M1 East Midlands Airport crash which appeared on TV. Without a moment's hesitation I felt that for some reason, perhaps a malfunctioning sixth sense, that Janet had been killed aboard that flight from Australia. I kept myself composed until I boarded the top deck of the bus back to the hospital when I started to cry. Another relapse had occurred.

During the times when my illness was at its worst I was very demanding to staff, particularly most often for instant attention regularly knocking the window of the nurse's station. This impatience was particularly heightened on Thursday's ward round, where I would constantly ask staff whether it was my turn to go into 'the room' and see the multi-disciplinary panel of doctors, social workers etc. I craved attention all the time.

I developed a notion that my bank account had been tampered with by some higher authorities (which included my mother for some reason). The balance would not reckon with what I had expected. As a result I told my mother off over the phone and had to apologise when I came to my senses.

To a certain extent I was aware from previous experience that the medication given was going to reduce my level of functioning so that my ability to initiate and maintain conversation would be reduced, my motivation (even to get out of bed in the morning) would diminish and that my running as a serious pastime would be put on the backburner once again. I did not want these side effects to occur so I tried to fight them off by being as active as I possibly could. I started reading novels (JD Salinger's 'Catcher in the Rye'), doing jigsaws, going out as much as possible and socializing with fellow patients on my own and other wards at every opportunity. However, as the length of my stay in hospital increased so did the level of my medication. My ability to tell jokes, even bad ones disappeared along with my extrovert personality. I was not just like my previous reserved self, I was very passive, being more of a spectator that a participant of a group conversation. Rising for breakfast became a chore in itself, let alone the early morning exercise therapy sessions I had taken part in earlier in my stay.

It was true, I had prompted the staff to give me my initial injection (due to my mental anguish and torture I was suffering at the time) but I was rather manipulated into the final increase in dosage (which doubled my previous dose) and instantaneously turned me into a relative zombie despite dispensing completely with my delusional thoughts. When my conscious thoughts returned to the real world, it removed the fast, exciting, though torturous world I had lived in before and replaced it with an ordinary, mundane, slow, predictable, tame and relatively harmless world.

Around early February, just three weeks before the voices diminished completely, it occurred to me that Valentine's Day was approaching and although my obsession for Janet was fading away I still felt it necessary to send her a card care of her former University tutor. After posting the card I phoned the lecturer to tell her what I had done, only to meet a naturally frosty and shocked response. As the medication increased however, I began to accept my present predicament, letting go of my obsessions and becoming more patient and less demanding on the hospital ward.

It was quite often the case that the arrival of a seriously ill new admission to the ward would bring everybody down low in mood because it often meant having to put up with their anti social and delusional behaviour which many of us felt we had overcome.
I began to feel at home on the ward from early March onwards and had built up some strong friendships. My best friend on the ward was Paul who was receiving ECT and Lithium treatment for his illness. He had suffered severe post traumatic symptoms after leaving the Territorial Army in the early 80's. I was quite shocked when he told me

that ECT treatment was a means of electronically inducing something similar to an epileptic fit in order to block out a depressive state. The problem was it tended to block out recent memory span as well (usually temporarily).

Another friend was a graduate in Chemistry who had suffered his initial breakdown in the early 70's and who had traveled the country, going in and out of hospital every few years.

Philip was another friend who lived with his mother and who had come into hospital for observation to fine tune his level of medication. He tended to look back on his life, like many people on the ward, in a fatalistic way, stating that his life was now a tragedy and that he was a failure as many people with mental illness also feel. The experience of mental illness can often be so embarrassing that, in addition to society stigmatizing mentally ill people, mentally ill people stigmatise themselves.

A few of the younger patients who I felt were very "street cred" weasled out of me that I was a virgin and with utter contempt for my integrity offered a whip round so that I could lose my innocence in one night of cheap passion in Balsall Heath. Obviously I refused.

However, I did not refuse the role of errand boy smuggling whiskey into the outside hospital grounds in return for a little money to buy some chocolate. In other respects I was more conformative with the hospital regime.

The occupational therapy sessions were interesting and stimulating. My favourite being the 7.30am exercise therapy session which I was able to motivate myself to take part in before the psychiatric medication took its hold. Unlike the patronizing style of the exercise sessions at the previous hospital in Leicester, these sessions were a serious attempt to push each patient as hard as possible with an instructor as demanding as any running coach I had had. The same instructor ironically ran a relaxation course. The deep breathing techniques I learned from these sessions have enabled me to keep well for many years since this relapse.

One therapy session I did find inappropriate was called 'Social and Dancing'. No contemporary dance techniques were taught. I found the Waltz useful but dances like the Military Two Step went out decades ago. However, one good outcome of my first session was that I met my former girlfriend Lara by walking up to her and asking her to dance with me. It was a short but sweet friendship. She was on a secure ward because she had attempted suicide but she did not seem depressed in my company and despite being 'petite' was more than capable of looking after herself on a very hazardous ward. When I visited her ward I asked why all the chairs were bolted down, she said that before they were, she never walked about without looking behind her in case a table or chair was thrown. She packed me in when I was unable to see her for five days after she had moved to a rehabilitation hostel in Acocks Green. I was very upset but determined I was not going to make myself ill so I began to accept what had happened and switched off from it all.

By the time of my 24th birthday in late March I was no longer psychotic, paranoid or delusional and had made a "clinical recovery" with a medical formula that was considered satisfactory. The injection not only slowed down my thought processes so that they were in tune with reality, they also slowed down my metabolism and I increased my weight by 2 ¼ stones in two months. Inability to do intensive training also had a negative effect on my waistline which went from 32inches to 36inches over the same period. At a ward round at about this time, the multi-disciplinary team decided to present me with a choice. I was well enough to either go home or, to go to work from the ward on a trial basis, not both. The fact that I had become used to the homely environment of the hospital surroundings, tempered by my eagerness to get back to work, prompted me to plump for the latter option.

It did not take long for me to regret my decision (one working day). The slower nature of my thought processes magnified the tedious aspects of the job and even worse made the day drag more and more. My clock watching behaviour developed into an obsessional level as I willed each separate hour (and fraction of each hour) on. I reluctantly agreed to comply with the original plan to gradually increase the small number of hours each week to full time. But I felt trapped, the quality of my life had suddenly evaporated, as I spent the hours outside of work slumped either in bed or on the sofa. After a soul bearing session with the manager I handed in my notice and left in late July after just 13-months of service. By this time, I had been discharged from hospital. It only took a month of spending the daytime periods (because my brother was at work) on my own (I had no day centres to go to). I decided I needed an environment where I could mix with others to prevent myself vegetating and got my social worker to refer me to a social services psychiatric hostel in Small Heath.

PART FOUR

EYE WITNESS ACCOUNTS OF MY ILLNESS.

Philip was always the active one. Full of energy. He had no fear of the world around him. There was the time when he was on the swing in the garden. Backward and forwards he went, higher and higher. While at the top of the swing he decided to get off, so off he came and landed on his feet running.

Another time when he was on the beach at Charmouth we were building sandcastles. Philip decided he'd had enough so off he ran, and ran and ran – past all the people on the beach. He suddenly decided he did not know where he was and started to panic. Myself and his father Al had followed him so no harm came to him.

As he got older he continued his running. Through school first and then onto Birchfield Harriers followed by Sparkhill Harriers. Even at University this was Philip, studying and running.

My sister had informed me of Philip's illness while in Leicester. She told me not to be surprised at Philip's condition so I went round to see him. Even so, seeing Philip sitting in my sister's living room with his dressing gown on, staring blankly at the wall, I was taken aback. This certainly wasn't the lad I'd watched grow up. He looked aged, pale a blank expression across his face. His speech was so very slow when he did speak. Could the medication explain his slow action? I still don't know. The spark of life had gone out of

him. I tried to have a conversation but this proved fruitless. He would start to answer and then drift off to some other place.
My sister kept me informed of his progress over the next few weeks, he was improving but very slowly. On visiting again I noticed an improvement but it was very small. All his ambition had left him. On broaching the subject of Leicester, the University and his exams he seemed unwilling to speak, so I let the subject drop. In fact only on reading the original manuscript of the book did I find out exactly what happened all those years ago.

Months passed, Philip slowly improved to a standard where he could go out and face the world. I asked him if he would like to go fishing with my stepfather and myself and he said he would. But watching him sit on the river bank, it was the same Philip who sat in the house letting the world pass by without really participating. He showed little interest in the art of fishing – I would cast in for him, I would tell him what to look for in the was of a bite followed a little later by me reeling in and starting all over again. Philip could not concentrate at all as far as I could see so the fishing was not a success, but the day was nice and it was a chance to leave all my cares behind, if not so for Philip.

They say time is a healer, in Philip's case this is not quite true after a few years and one relapse Philip is somewhere near his old self, he is very active again in his life. He has married, something that seemed and impossibility back in those dark, distant days. He holds down a responsible job looking after people with similar problems to himself. But all of these things are only achieved with the aid of his medication. Philip visits us most weeks so we see the different stages of his medication. From the first few days after his injection, when he seems a little confused and struggles to concentrate to the following couple of weeks where he is his old self again, so full of enthusiasm and self confidence, to the last week where he slows down and starts to go back into his shell. Only for the whole cycle to start again.

I know this is not perfect but compared to how he was, sitting in the living room all those years ago, I could not ask for more.

By Ian Roberts, younger brother of my foster mother.

A Tutor's Memories.

I am embarrassed to admit that my memories of Philip's experiences eight years later are rather vague. I did not know him well, but had been his tutor for a short while two years earlier when his own tutor was away. I do remember his visit to Leicester in the summer of 1987 though. I was in the common room with some colleagues in the quiet days when the hectic activity of examinations is over, and the students had gone home. No doubt I was having a cup of tea to put off returning to my research work. A student who I vaguely recognized appeared, looking, I thought, for his tutor, who was himself away on holiday at the time. Since the visitor was evidently in some distress I agreed to see him, thinking that perhaps he was upset about examination results and needed some counseling. I don't recall the details of the discussion, but Philip remembers that I agreed to tell Janet of his problems. I know that I was conscious that he was very confused and unwell, and was grateful that he was receiving appropriate medical care. His student record card mentions his breakdown after exams, and his tutor comments that it must have affected his exam performance, since it was below the very good standard of his course work during the year. All the tutors who taught Philip agreed that he was a bright and hardworking student.

I remember much more clearly teaching Janet, who kept in touch with me for some years. I also remember she shared my concern for Philip, and that she was anxious that he would find her home address. In fact I believe that she raised this issue with me before Philip himself did, and she was particularly anxious about returning to Leicester to do an MA course. She did not want to be unkind to him, but thought it would not be helpful if he were able to 'pursue' her there. However she was concerned enough to want to know how he was, and it was sometimes difficult to satisfy her genuine concern without breaking Philip's confidences, particularly since she did not want him to know that I was in touch with her. For several years she sent me Christmas cards, and it is probably my fault that we are no longer in touch. Janet and I were both amateurs, trying to help a distressed young man, but way out of our depth in terms of medical knowledge. Under the circumstances I think we were lucky not to do him any harm.

My memory of the 'Valentine card' event is also rather hazy. I was probably at the time preoccupied by the break up of my own marriage, and increasing responsibilities at work. I know that Philip phoned me quite frequently at this time, often with very little to say, but in evident distress and wanting to make contact. These phone calls often lasted well over an hour, and at one time were about weekly (usually on Tuesday evenings!) He didn't especially want to talk about Janet, but about his experience at University and his difficulty holding down a job which he felt challenged him. At work the next day I often found he had spent an equal amount of time on the phone to another colleague the same evening, so there was obviously a desperate need to talk. I was acutely aware of my own ignorance and tried just to be a listening ear, fearful of making suggestions which might be misinterpreted.

Since then the phone calls have become less frequent, shorter and much more focused. I was thrilled when Philip invited me to his wedding, and was only prevented from attending by a last minute family 'crisis'. I've been glad to see Philip on a couple of his recent visits to Leicester, and have been impressed by his support of his wife in her recent illness.

Since my first encounter with Philip I have experienced considerable stress in my own life, and my awareness of my own fragility has made me more tolerant. As a student Philip was always something of a misfit and a loner, but I am very conscious of the waste his illness has caused and to which he refers. I admire tremendously both his honesty and his courage in acknowledging the problems, and finding ways of coping with them. I hope he will continue to keep in touch, and I look forward to following his progress. I certainly don't regret having 'got involved' and I wish him all the best for the future.

Catherine Waddams, April 1995.

My first reaction to Philip's illness was of utter shock and disbelief. This couldn't be happening again, like it did to his mother. I remember as a young girl visiting his mother in Hollymore (psychiatric hospital) on Sunday afternoons with my Gran. On one occasion she had been put in a straight-jacket and was in a padded cell. That incident has stayed with me all my life. Although his mother was violent, Philip never was.

I've had Philip since he was thirteen-months and although he calls me Mum, he really is my cousin and is also my mother's sister's child. For the first few years I had to take him to clinics and hospitals for one test and another. We were told at one stage that he would struggle through main stream school so when he made it to University I really couldn't believe it. I am so proud of Philip and I know he has been through an awful experience and has come through it. He has a good job caring for others and he enjoys it. One thing I can say about Philip is that he is a fighter and he will fight for as long as he has to.

Jessica Ruffle (Mum), Foster Mother and Cousin (i.e. my mother's sister's daughter)

It was a perfect summer evening. I was contentedly working on my allotment when I realized that something was developing. A friend had come with a message that Philip was ill in Leicester.
The next morning we drove to the hospital. That in itself was awful. We were unprepared, no map, no street guide and to add to our problems, any one we asked for guidance could not help.
When we did get to the hospital we found that Philip was very ill. The first doctor we spoke to gave us a clear description of the illness, in layman's terms, of how it could be controlled, and gave us back our hope.

The next year was a year of frustration as he would improve and then deteriorate.

I hoped he would stay at home until he fully recovered. But he wanted his independence and quickly moved into a flat with his brother Paul.

Paul started to complain about Philip's behaviour which we put down to their usual bouts of sparring. We did not realize that having come off his medication, his illness had returned. The good part was that Philip did, and sought treatment himself.

This time his illness was more pronounced. I felt he was more disturbed, or was he just talking more? He was quite pleased that he had not been fooled by their television subterfuge that was aimed at him and other patients.

I expect I will always worry that he may have another dark period, but at least we now know there is a way back.

In 1987 I thought I had lost a son, it's nice to have him back.

Albert Ruffle (Foster Father)

Commentary on the Eye Witness Accounts of my Illness.

Sometimes it is easy to forget how debilitated I was at one stage of my illness and the first account by Ian Roberts reminds me of how I must have appeared to others just after leaving hospital. It is one thing to not feel completely well, it is quite another to perceive how that must appear to other people.

Ian also draws some useful comparisons of how I appeared before my breakdown. I had particular close contact with Ian in the period immediately before my illness, visiting him and his wife Annette weekly during holiday periods between University academic terms. I still keep in regular contact with him.

When I received my former University Tutor's contribution to my book I read its contents with great anticipation. What I was surprised about was the extent to which Janet kept in contact with her tutor in the period after I graduated and the extent to which their concern for me lead to me being a recurrent topic of conversation between them. I was initially slightly angry and upset about what I regarded to be the ambiguous attitude of Janet towards me. She wanted to know how I was but did not want me to know she was still in touch with our mutual tutor. A bit like trying to have your cake and eat it, as I thought at the time. But now I feel that as Janet has a concern for my well being which is tempered by a genuine fear she has of contact with me, which is not only based on the poor impression she formed of me at University, but on the serious nature of my diagnosis which has helped reinforce this impression and ruled out even a pen friend relationship. She would not trust me as far as she could throw me and that would not be far.

I had reservations about my tutor's reference to me as a 'misfit' but on reflection I must have seemed like that to many observers and would regard it as an accurate term because I had reservations at the time about bowing to peer group pressure and when I decided that I wanted to be one of the 'in crowd' I was clueless how to go about it. However, I would have regarded myself more of a 'Maverick and loner' that a 'misfit and loner' at the time. I find my tutor's opinion of my academic ability very flattering and feel pleased she has not regretted her contact with me since University.

My foster mother's account of my illness is very much about the shock of seeing her worst nightmare confirmed, namely the diagnosis of her son with the same illness as my natural mother of which she has vivid haunting memories of seeing her in a straight-jacket. Fortunately, due to the development of medication as a means of controlling the illness, she did not have to suffer the ordeal of seeing me in a straight-jacket. However, the sight of me when she first visited at Leicester General with my Dad was harrowing enough for her. She admires the way I have been able to piece together my life. Since my illness and we both had had a mutual foreboding of my developing a lifelong dependence – i.e. being unable to assert my adult role and needing lifelong care in a family setting.

My Dad has always been proud of me and has never been short of a word of congratulation or reassurance. He must have felt I was set up for life when I gained my place at University. He was very frustrated by the periods of illness and set backs he had to endure. He seems to be very wary of not being lulled into a false sense of security by presuming everything is okay because I am stabilized on a particular medication. He appreciates how much of a struggle it is for me to remain well and realizes how vulnerable I am to the possibility of relapse.

PART FIVE.

REHABILITATION.

My descent from a relatively autonomous life in the community to dependence was started by my illness which in turn initiated a chain of negative thoughts and doubts about my own ability. Firstly I resigned from my job then, gave up my accommodation and finally lost the will to thoroughly look after myself. After 13-months of full-time work I had known what it was like to be a member of the 'rat race', like a mouse trying to ascend a spinning wheel. I had gained little from my experience of living away from my parents and with my brother and my job had become a dead end. So I thought – why should I bother, why not take life easy and instead of making things happen as I used to, let things take care of themselves. As a result of this attitude my personal hygiene deteriorated, as did the quality of my diet and my days, which once seemed so full, were now empty with long periods of inactivity.

Losing your job is accompanied by the loss of your role and your status. Suddenly you are a dependent. It is not long before you lose your confidence and by the time I arrived at the hostel this process was at an advanced stage. Conditions were now ripe for the development of a less responsible attitude to myself and others. This attitude was not specifically attributable to me alone but was also very much an adoption by me of already established values of the residents' subculture. At least I had a peer group.

Such an abdication of responsibility was soon apparent to the hostel in Birmingham, where I was now to live after an assessment period, for nearly 12-months. Just as the staff gained a clear picture of me, so I obtained an insight into the comparative deficiencies in the care they provided.

There was little attempt at therapeutic intervention and people who were exhibiting challenging behaviour were often seen as attention seeking and dealt with in a largely unsympathetic manner.

Much of the time was spent by staff in meetings and their availability and time was limited which tended to store up resentment and anxieties in certain residents to such an extent that therapeutic intervention at a later stage was more difficult. I was resident for a period of four-months before anybody attempted to help me tidy my room and it was at this stage I was first introduced to any progress report on what they had decided were my areas of need. Furthermore, I was not involved in the assessment process and no work was done to deal with or probe the underlying insecurities that lingered from both my periods of mental illness. This rudderless and uncoordinated pattern of care provision was not necessarily complete hindrance and I was able to use my stay as one long period of respite. It may have hampered others however, some of whom may have had less potential to recover from mental illness and who needed more than just respite.

The days were now empty with long periods of total inactivity. Everything that had previously given my life structure and something to get up for had now gone and the boredom made me dwell on the side effects of the medication which seemed stronger during periods of inactivity than in more active periods.

It did not take long for me to develop a UB40 (unemployed) sleep pattern of going to bed between one and two o'clock in the morning to get up at midday. The earliest each week that I had to get up was for the 11am fire drill on Monday mornings and even that was a chore.

My diet quickly lost its variation until it became little more than a succession of fry-ups. Furthermore, I considered it both wise and cost effective to eat less regularly (only twice a day so that I could lose weight).

In addition to this I had a tendency to lie down on my bed and drop off to sleep which meant my clothes always looked creased.

I had a particularly sadistic sense of humour at the time and a favourite activity of mine was to mimics other residents less fortunate than myself. This encouraged a regular wrestling match with one of the residents who was the butt of one of my jibes. On another occasion I was almost beaten up by a potentially violent resident who had a South African accent that provided an 'impersonation' opportunity which was too good to miss. I picked at weaknesses in peoples characters like a child picks scabs.

There was one tragic character who had lost both his parents at a formative age and had been so ill he had failed to develop a complete male physique. He had lost all his teeth around the same time and sounded very muffled and unclear. The staff had to ration his DSS money because otherwise it would be spent on huge quantities of cigarettes with no supplies of food as a result.

Another resident had also been at University and had an unfortunate experience with a relationship with a woman. He was extremely reserved but had a dry sense of humour and liked to play Chinese Whispers and the occasional practical joke on people.

One of the residents had "extreme tardic dyskinesia", which are facial tics which resulted in involuntary movements in his cheeks. This had been caused by years of taking Lithium to alleviate the symptoms of his mental illness.

A certain Polish resident was nicknamed "Jesus" on his arrival due to appearance of his long, unkempt hair and beard. However, he had his hair cut and looked far more presentable after a short while. The illness had slowed down his movements so they had become laboured and his speech droned. He was very quiet and sat around looking into space most of the time.

It was interesting when we went on a hostel holiday (the first of two holidays with the hostel) to a place near Fort William in Scotland. A male member of staff and ex-paratrooper dominated proceedings. He took us out on an excursion one day which was a four – five hour round journey with barely a 45 minute stay at our destination.

When I look back I can also appreciate that most of the time a majority of the staff were quite supportive of me during times of indecision and uncertainty and I miss a few of them greatly.

The biggest turning point in my life was meeting my future wife. At first I thought she was a visiting nurse and found out instead she was a resident. That night I sat with her and it did not take me more than a few days to realize that she was the most polite and considerate person I had ever met. It was not long before we were constantly in one another's company. A romantic courtship ensued.

It was not long before I started, by shopping with her, to emulate her varied and nutritionally balanced diet and began to eat more regularly. She often washed and ironed my clothes and not surprisingly insisted that I no longer slept in my clothes (a habit that gradually became less frequent). Furthermore, my days became full of activity as I accompanied her to visit places all over the Midlands. In return I offered my 'wife to be' the emotional support she needed and bullied her into doing things she previously lacked the confidence to do.

For a short period we moved into a dodgy private flat offered by a landlord in Moseley and were bailed out and allowed to return to the hostel. After just six weeks on the waiting list we were offered a ground floor flat by a reputable housing association and in October 1990 moved in.

My wife over the period of our relationship has given me back the sense of responsibility I had lost. In return I feel that I may have helped her become a more confident person. She has done more than anybody else to ensure that I have successfully held down a work career for four years by taking care of most of the cooking, washing and cleaning. I live in a pleasant environment because my wife is a real home maker. Unfortunately the hole in my wallet seems to have got larger and larger since I met her. We have been through some rough times and sometimes bicker frequently but I feel that is a sign of a well balanced relationship where the balance of power seems to shift round a central point.

With a stable home and work environment I have been able to achieve many things. In April, 1993 I successfully completed the London Marathon raising 900 pounds for the Midlands region of a mental health charity, NSF. I have been Social Secretary of Northfield Branch Labour Party for three consecutive years and am currently Political Education Officer. I have also served for two years as School Governor on the Governing Body of West Heath Junior and Infant Schools. Finally, I have successfully taken up the flute and have made slow but steady progress. The process of getting up for work every morning imposed strict parameters on my sleep pattern, furthermore I was accountable both at work and at home for the use of my time. Over a period of years this encouraged a more mature and less childlike attitude to my responsibilities to myself and to others. The weekly act of Christian worship gave me a moral and ethical basis for continuing the newly adopted lifestyle and reinforced this psychological ageing process. Mixing with people at work (and in my social life) who did not have mental health difficulties promoted a process of normalization which underlined my gradual change in attitude to life in general.

Despite times of great motivation there are times when I have lingered in bed longer than I should have. The more I laid there the more depressed I feel but I always snap out of it when I finally get up. To lead a successful and enjoyable life there is often a need for every two steps forward to require a consolidating step back.

PART SIX.

MY QUEST TO FIND WORK.

Finding a job is not easy at the best of times without having to overcome the prejudice of employers towards people who have had nervous breakdowns.

From my graduation to my first decent job with the Education Department of Birmingham City Council there was a three year period of job hunting during which, at a conservative estimate, I applied for about two to three hundred jobs.

There is not only a specific stigma directed against people who have suffered mental illness, there is a general discrimination against disabled people as a whole and a misconception over the definition disabled. There is legislation to uphold the rights and prevent discrimination to disabled people but this is not always enforced. Larger organizations have taken on board many if not all of the criteria of equal opportunities practice. However, smaller organizations still adhere to ad hoc recruitment procedures and as a result discrimination is more widespread in this sector.

If you mention the word *disabled* to most people their first thought is to think of someone in a wheelchair or someone who is blind, deaf or has cerebral palsy. However, this definition excludes people with more latent disabilities such as multiple sclerosis and in mental illness especially schizophrenia who may need support in finding and keeping a job but who nevertheless have a valuable contribution to make to any potential employer and indeed society as a whole.

I have encountered some employers who have had the effrontery to tell me off for being a time waster despite the time and expense I have taken to fill in application forms and make the bus journeys. Other employers feel sorry for me when I mention my illness but this sympathy does not extent to providing me with a chance to prove myself and instead makes them consider the job too stressful for me (in a patronizing manner).

I found continued rejection particularly when no 'honest' feedback was offered, made me valued myself less. The reduction in confidence coming across at subsequent interviews making it less and less likely I would get a job. Society values those who are given access to work by giving them access to goods and services through their wage packet. Being unemployed and harbouring feelings of inferiority due to my disability made me feel like a second class citizen. And made me wonder whether I would ever (via a wage packet) be entitled to a better quality of living. I will now give a potted history of my quest for work.

In the months leading up to my first illness I had had some partial success and had gained a couple of second interviews. Then it seemed only a matter of time before I would hit the jackpot and be able to continue the independent life I had at University.

I counted myself out of contention from the high powered graduate type jobs on discharge from

Leicester General. Instead I applied for jobs that required lower academic entry standards.

I adopted a twin strategy, some employers I told of my illness, others I did not. I used what leeway the application forms would allow me to cover up my breakdown.

The question most often asked was why is a graduate like you applying for a menial job like this? It was at this stage I revealed the nature of the illness I had suffered only to be confronted by a U-turn in the attitude of the interview panel. From being considered over qualified for a particular job, the job so I was told, would be too stressful for me.

To make things worse the medication sapped the animated look from my face and slowed my thoughts down to an extent that I found it difficult to give off-the-cuff answers to the less predictable interview questions.

In December 1987 I started a training scheme at the Employment Rehabilitation Centre. This was a Department of Employment project aimed at assessing and training people with a wide range of disabilities. Government cuts however had reduced the average length of stay to such a degree that it was barely able to assess people let alone meet the training needs of clients. In the end my stay was just seven to eight weeks. All I had gained was a school leaver's type of certificate with competence headings for very basic skills. To put it another way, it would barely complement my degree certificate in my present folder.

When I joined Washwood Heath Job Club in April/May 1988 I had to complete the mandatory village idiot's course on how to look for work in return for free postage, free papers and the use of a phone.   When I obtained a job as a postal filing clerk in June 1988 it did not take long for the euphoria to die down and to be replaced by a deepening resentment towards the menial nature of the job. As I explained earlier, I had to resign from this job to make a full recovery in my level of functioning after traumatic illness.

There was a period of about six months after my resignation when I returned to my quest for full time work whilst living in residential accommodation. I volunteered to go on a training course to develop typing and office skills. It soon became clear to even the most persistent instructor that I would never make the grade as a typist and they had little else, at that time, to offer in terms of recognized office qualifications. Furthermore, they were not providing me with the practical work experience placement required after the initial six weeks of training. So I decided to sacrifice my extra 10.00 pounds a week and resigned from the course.

Eventually I had good fortune.   I attended an interview for a low paid administration clerk at a warehouse in Erdington and was asked just one difficult question at the interview – Are you in good

health?   During the short hesitation in answering the question various thoughts entered my head. Do they want my definition of my own good health (a perfectly healthy individual taking prescribed medication like millions of others) or their definition where I would divulge all?   I decided in the end that it was worth taking a risk and responded yes. Even if I was dismissed for being economical with the truth, I would have gained some valuable experience, not to mention money in the meantime.   They phoned three hours later to tell me that I had got the job.
The job was like a stock controllers 'mate' and I only worked there long enough to learn the basics of stock taking (cookers, home fires and camp equipment) with a smattering of knowledge to bluff my way through basic phone enquiries., manual stock, record adjustment and computerised stock control (where I messed up nearly all the records).

My big break came when I was informed in mid-August (1990) of my interview for a job as a clerical assistant in the Education Department of the City Council for an application I had sent off three months earlier. I was to find on arrival at the interview that half the people had found suitable work, which narrowed it down to me and three other candidates. During the interview I admitted my original illness (but left out anything about my relapse) and was hardly able to string two sentences together for the less predictable questions. I resigned myself to the rejection heap so was ecstatic to receive a phone call the very next day offering me the job. My mood became deflated when I found that a query had arisen on my medical form and I would require a full medical. After a few nights of poor sleep I passed the medical with a green light.

I started the job with the wrong attitude and was over concerned due to my previous reactions to stress and not to push myself to hard. I soon developed a good idea of the office workload and made work last as long as possible. I eased off too much and when I realized the need to try harder it was difficult to shake off the mediocre first impression I had created for myself. In retrospect I feel that a career in clerical work was unsuitable for me because my attention to detail was often poor. Nevertheless, the job did get me into a habit of getting up early most mornings (despite of the usual side effects from medication) and my level of self confidence increased. The most important skill I improved upon was my telephone manner. However, in many ways I was fed up and due to the cuts and ever growing competition for council clerical jobs in higher grades, I concluded I was in a dead end job. The turning point for my next career move proved to be a council course provided by a private company called "Tragic but Brave" called "Career Development for People with Disabilities" Before this course I had considered doing a part time post graduate thesis in an economic history subject at Birmingham University. The disabled providers of this course persuaded me to pursue a secondary plan I had had to apply for jobs in the care field especially mental health where my user insight would offer organizations with a provider of care who had insight and empathy with the clients. The early scare to my future job security that was temporarily posed by even tighter council budgets and the move of schools to not the service of the council (by being grant maintained) gave me a further spur and kick started me into looking for another job.

Care work provided me with a chance to have direct contact with a client, not just talking from an office at the end of a telephone. I found out about a City & Guilds course being offered at my local college (Bournville College of FE) and it became clear that I would need a placement so I plumped for a nursing home run by the National Schizophrenia Fellowship in Winson Green where I had previously had a job rejection. With the help of the volunteer services of West Birmingham Health Authority it was agreed that during my weekends off (from the office job I still had) I would work on Sundays for between four to seven hours. I built such a good relationship with the residents that on the occasional week I turned up on a Saturday, the residents would think it was a Sunday. Having to do assignments for my college work, which were largely based on building relationships with individual residents, helped me to evaluate my work and to learn more from input I was making as well as providing opportunities to provide simple, social college based theories to practice. I treated all residents, in one sense as though they were fellow patients on the ward in an attempt to speak at their level without patronizing them. Much of my work in taking the residents out and in spending individual time with each of them on a one-to-one basis added to the work done by staff which due to the routine nature of many of their duties, they sometimes found difficult to fit in. I made such a big impact in such a short time that I was offered the post of care officer at the rehabilitation wing of the home after just six months as a volunteer.

PART SEVEN.

MY EXPERIENCE AS A MENTAL HEALTH CARER.

I found that there were many differences between the roles of care officer and volunteer. It was easy to be popular with the residents as a befriender, there was no need to challenge their behaviour or to get them to do things they did not feel like doing. As a care officer it was often necessary to try and re-establish , as well as to build and maintain therapeutic carer relationships, when you got on the wrong side of a particular resident. Furthermore, the quality of the of the relationship between myself and the people I cared for, was not just an end in itself, but now a means of gaining the necessary leverage in motivating residents to co-operate with mutually agreed plans of care.

Initially there was a tendency for me as a user of mental health services, to feel that I had a novel or unique approach to care and it took a while for me to appreciate the many and varied skills that other people from different backgrounds can bring to the care of residents and that it was the ability to work as a team rather than as autonomous individuals that was needed to reach the overall objectives of care provision. I found very quickly that, no one member of staff got on well with every single resident and that many of them had different favourites who would find it easier to motivate certain residents.

During my experience as a care officer I had my fair share of personality clashes and one cause was differing personal care philosophies held between staff members. Such differences were not always settled with the formal framework of handover, supervision sessions and staff meetings, with feelings being vented in the form of work place gossip and backstabbing. A staff away day did much to solve what were once difficult staff problems.

An aspect of my work which took a while to master, was the paperwork. It took a while to develop a routine, so that I could document the health and care of each resident, as well as the care services they received. By getting the opportunity to conduct resident reviews I became better at formulating plans of care for them as well as learning to liaise with other health care professional, CPNs, GPs, psychologists, social workers, relatives etc.

The full time nature of my role as a care officer enabled me to obtain more materials for assignments for college and I completed my City & Guilds in Community Care Practice in July 1993.

I have gained more job satisfaction in care than in any other type of work because of the larger scope to take on responsibility and use initiative. This is particularly the case of the more independent wing of the nursing home where I worked. Because of staff shortages and the resultant lack of supervision I have had to work very much under my own steam learning basic time management and prioritization skills. I find that working for a charity has increased my level of motivation to a higher level that I have had in any other job.

The shift pattern, at times, could be stressful, with up to 26 hours at a time away from home due to the nature of 'sleep-ins' There were times when I did feel stressed out and I reacted by ensuring I made the time to fit in my breaks so that I had the opportunity to sit down, relax and unwind. I also ensued that the shift pattern did not lead to a deterioration in my diet. I was particularly prone to 'stress reactions' in the period of the week before my injection was due (I often counted the days and hours until my depot when feeling stressed). On the other hand I also found it a struggle to function at work in the four or five day period immediately following my injection and felt slightly less 'on-the-ball' than usual. I responded to this by bringing my Procyclodine tablets to work in the hope they would give me a 'buzz'.

At times when I did feel 'stressed' it was difficult to be 'responsive' to residents. However a rest day, a weekend off or annual leave often recharged my batteries so that I became more amiable on my return to work.

Work was often hectic, particularly when many residents were competing for my attention at one time. It is at such times that I reflected on my demanding behaviour in hospital and felt more able to empathize with the way ward staff responded to me then.

During my time as a volunteer and in the early part of my time as a care officer I had an unrealistic 'whiter than white' image of the residents and it has taken me a long time to realize that residents 'are not as innocent' as I once thought, being as capable as anybody else in their ability to manipulate (staff and other residents). It was difficult to initially intervene when challenging or awkward behaviour occurred.

It was very hard not to have occasional negative feelings towards residents who change their minds after staff have put themselves out to meet an earlier request or who became verbally abusive and (occasionally) physically threatening. However, if negative thoughts, however justified, are allowed to

dwell, there was a detrimental effect on your morale and subsequently to your motivation to be an effective carer.

The residents I used to care for have spent a large number of years on the long term wards psychiatric wads of All Saints Hospital and had to a certain extent become 'institutionalized'. The emphasis of the care was to provide 'a home for life' for each resident and even in the more independent wing of the project, there was a resident-led approach with no overall deadlines by which the residents needed to be moved on to suitable alternative accommodation. In my experience there has only been one person who has successfully moved on to a more independent project.

The fact that I have a successful change of career is a positive outcome of my illness which is in contrast to a view I once held where I saw my breakdown as a tragic turning point in my life.

Furthermore, the job allowed me to use at least some of the skills I gained at University and I felt a respected and valued member of a team at Latimer House.

During my first four months at Latimer Nursing Home I worked as a night shift Care Officer. This was a very unusual experience because I had to stay awake between the hours of 8pm. until 8am. Whilst on duty, if I had any pressing engagements during the day I could, occasionally, go without sleep for up to 24 hours. Some nights could be literally non stop for most of the period but usually there was a lull in activity between 12.30am and 5am during which time I could write letters or read.

Whilst working these shifts I learned to concentrate and work when feeling either run down and tired and because I did so many hours in a short concentrated period of the week it seemed as though I had more days off. Even now, if I lose track of time late at night I can end up staying up in the early hours without feeling tired.

I felt I was getting nowhere fast in my job at Latimer (Due to lack of promotional prospects) and over a period of three to six months around the middle of 1994 I made more of an effort to find another job in the mental health field.

I made a third attempt at getting a job at South Birmingham Rehabilitation Unit (also run by the same charity, the NSF) this time for the more senior post of Senior Care Officer. It was a difficult interview and I was uncertain how I had done.

I was amazed when at about 10am. On November 30th I got a phone call to tell me I had got the job.

The fact I had obtained the post meant that I had been promoted within the NSF and between hearing that good news and actually starting the job on January 2nd, 1995, I felt better about myself for a more sustained period than in all my life.

However, on starting the job I started to worry about it from day one, over eager to make the right impression, afraid of making mistakes and allowing uncertainty that comes with any new job to eat away at my confidence.

I have now accepted that making mistakes is an inevitable part of the learning process. I developed a familiarity with the routine and philosophy of the project and, along with plenty of assurance from my supervisor, I was able to rebuild my confidence. Despite the job being stressful and feeling stretched at times, I also felt I had grown as an individual and therefore became better at time management, prioritization and attention to detail amongst other things.

The project catered for people who have suffered from mental illness and who showed potential for looking after themselves in the community, with a maximum stay of two-years. The degree of support they got at their next accommodation depended on progress made at the unit and an assessment was made of their progress throughout and at the end of their stay. Residents were encouraged to do as much for themselves as possible in the hope that they would be empowered enough to control their own lives. Ultimate goals at rehabilitation were dependent on the identified needs of each of the residents which varied according to the individual. Support, for instance was offered in such areas as medication (with the ultimate goal of self medication), shopping (with a menu plan to help compile shopping lists), cooking (opportunities were provided for people to broaden their cooking skills), domestic skills (namely room cleaning and laundry) and so on. This was fitted in along with other activities (such as day centres or other rehabilitation activity) into a weekly programme where residents were encouraged to enter their own appointments (eg. doctors and dentists etc.) After thorough consultation assessment, (including each resident) during the first four weeks of their stay, the residents needs were identified and care plans drawn up with each resident. Most of the care plans had short term goals where the resident is offered support in an area of rehabilitation from staff. The long term goal of the plan usually offered less or no support.

I found the medication induction course difficult (a course set up for unqualified senior staff so they could dispense medication from medidoses, safely) and then found myself in a role encouraging residents to take tablets at strict times, an area I wasn't tested on during my rehabilitation due to my total reliance on a depot injection.

One or two residents taught me cooking skills, but were lacking in other skills which proves why you need to consult and support every resident as an individual. This was done through key worker sessions once a week.

Residents were also encouraged to enter into their own folders and to monitor their own medication charts by signing the medication charts.

The main difference from the previous job was that residents were encouraged by persuasion to set their own boundaries and goals and the carer's job is often to sell ideas to the residents which they adopt when they settle into the community (ideas such as sensible diet, sleep pattern, medication etc.)

I look at the fortnightly supervision sessions that took place with a mixture of anxiety and relief. Relief in the sense that I had a forum to discuss my worries concerning my role, and anxiety because I had to take on board constructive criticism. I began to learn how to take such criticism without taking it too personally.

In my new role as Senior Care Officer I was responsible (amongst other things) for the implementation of care. This could not be done in isolation, even if you were a key worker to a particular resident, you wanted others to implement care plans properly in your absence. This required a great deal of teamwork and the need to set up appropriate meetings and discussions with other staff and other mental health professionals.

There was a great deal of difference between the care of Latimer Nursing Home and South Birmingham Rehabilitation Unit. At Latimer I was very much doing things for people whereas in the other job staff often asked residents to do more for themselves. Secondly, at the unit I worked with younger residents nearer my own age as well as dispensing medication. I was sometimes left overnight to look after the residents as the person in charge (with the keys) and consequently I then led the handover the next morning.

I am very aware that I was a role model (as well as other staff) for the residents to look up to and I tried to set an example by sharing and looking presentable on duty. I found it hard to be a role model because of once seeing other patients on the ward as my peer group, when I was previously ill myself. I had initial difficulty in keeping a "professional distance" from residents. When I was ill I regarded the nurses and doctors on the wards of Highcroft Hospital and Leicester General as very much parental figures with me acting out the child role (transactional analysis theory). This may be partly because I like to conform and found it difficult (due to my passive nature) to challenge the decisions that were taken on my behalf. When I lost my independence of living away from home at university (after my first breakdown) I came home to act out the child like figure due to the way in which the illness sapped my level of functioning, thereby reducing any confidence or any feelings of self esteem and self worth that I had had. To conclude, I like the fact that I am now utilizing many of the written and verbal communication skills I gained at University and now have a greater sense of self worth and esteem.

CHAPTER EIGHT.

FROM WRITING A DISSERTATION TO PUTTING TOGETHER A THESIS: MY POSTGRADUATE JOURNEY.

Overcoming the barriers.

Having attained a valuable role working as a full time professional carer in the mental health system I was still somehow unfulfilled. The nature of this yearning became apparent on my first visit for seven years to Leicester University in 1995. I cried when I walked past the Porter's Lodge on campus. It was clear I had not dealt with all the painful issues of the past. A major part of my inability to move on was the feeling that I had not fulfilled my potential and that somehow I had wasted my degree education. I also felt that despite my degree education that I did not have the respect of managers at work. I yearned for the opportunity once more to prove myself. My illness had prevented me saying a proper goodbye to my mates. I was engaged at the time in the first attempt to capture my life in the form of an auto-biography in which I was to define my life in terms of my mental health issues.

Whilst on campus I met up with Dr. Catherine Waddams (formerly Dr. Price who had once been Janet's tutor). She agreed at this meeting to make a contribution to my book and we also talked about the latest developments in our lives. She had been through a difficult time and identified closely with the issues of traumatic change that I had been through. She took a particular interest in my psychotherapy. I often dwelt on negative feelings that I had where I felt that my mental health issues had debilitated me as a person who had once been intelligent. I was desperate to capture that bright spark within. I also wanted to move from a job where I was being systematically bullied. The bullying led me to devalue any contribution I could make in a future job.

My solution was to improve my confidence by attaining a postgraduate qualification. The prospect of study also seemed a good way of dealing with the loneliness of separation from my wife. I identified a course on which I wanted to enroll. This was a Postgraduate Diploma in Economic Development and Policy. The choice was difficult because I could not identify a job from which I could move on to with this qualification. However, I believed that studying was about improving my confidence and that my background in Economics was a critical strength on which this course would build.

After being refused a regular fixed day off each week to study on a part time basis by my boss, I temporarily gave up on the idea. However, six months later I sold the idea to my manager by saying that I would work weekends in return for a regular day off in the week.

A final hurdle to overcome, for students with mental health issues, at that time before the implementation of the Disability Discrimination Act, was to get written permission from my psychiatrist before I could enroll. This precondition has been a known stumbling block to some people with mental health issues getting into University. Fortunately I had spent years nurturing the trust of my psychiatrist and he gladly gave his written permission.

It was clear that if I were to juggle a part time Postgraduate qualification with a full time job that there had to be more to study than getting a qualification. Study would intentionally become a new hobby.   The process of learning would hopefully stimulate me and enrich most aspects of my life.

However, before I could go ahead the bank would need to lend me about 1000 pounds for each of the two years I studied. Fortunately, they agreed.

My Aunt's Advice.

Before finally signing on the dotted line I consulted the person whom I respected most, Aunt Rene.

I explained to my aunt that I was not sure that the study would necessarily guarantee me a good job and it was a bit of a risk. She was a woman who had visited me in hospital at my worst and bearing this in mind what she said next surprised me.

She stated that she did not want me to get to her age and regret what might have been. If I could take advantage of the opportunities then at least when I got to her age I would not regret missed chances. Even if I were to fail she said, at least I would have tried.

Aunt Rene died three-months later and it took me five years to finally express how I felt about that and what it meant to me. She had died at the age of 75 from a massive stroke. Sitting down during the Christmas break five years later the words came to me in a poem called "Away in a Manger (Part Two)". It went as follows:

No one could be found as a genuine helper
No room in the community shelter,
No stable but a revolving door,
Three men had visited their assessment,
According to the law
And his angel had deserted him once more,
To a stale smelling asylum
The only shelter,
A lonely man slumped on a bed,
 That he called his helter skelter,
No visiting this place of the living dead,

An Aunt called Rene through groceries she sifts,
From what she pulled out she bore him gifts,
An apple, milk and biscuits,
A baby he had once lain, in swaddling sheets,
His boasted second coming they did not greet,
She sat as he cried, his conception was overdue,
That mad as he could be,
He could have feelings too,
She suspended his hand and it quivered a lot,

That's the way it is she said when your nerves are shot,
I sat in the church as her eulogy was read,
It was not that bad but a great deal went unsaid
And I told my brother the missing plot,
Then he said she had told him before she had died,
That returning home from that visit she had cried.

Dedicated to Rene Somerville 1921 -1995.

My First Year.

At the age of 31, in September, 1996 after nine years of absence from higher education I enrolled on a Postgraduate Diploma in Economic Development and Policy at the Centre for Urban and Regional Studies at the University of Birmingham.
What felt very strange to me when I strolled round 'Fresher's Fayre' was that I had experienced the students here as very different from the time I had been a student in the mid-1980. Were these students different or, without realizing it, had I changed? There seemed to be an hysterical excitement about the atmosphere and I decided that, with the twin commitments of full time work and part time study, I could not join up to many things.

The only society I joined was AngSoc. (The Anglican Society). My time within this religious community over the next eight years was not only an important part of my social life on campus but the rich fellowship I received helped to redefine how positive fellowship could be.

I remember vividly walking into my first lecture for over nine years. I was transfixed with excitement. The lecturer was Dr. Barbara Smith and she was facilitating a course entitled 'The Economy and Society: Interpreting Change'. The teaching style was fairly 'old school' and she read from a thick was of sheets that made up the hand out for each session. What was good was that she encouraged questions and towards the end of the morning tried to chair a debate.

Barbara had supervised over a hundred doctorate students and her unstinting service was to later earn her an OBE. Her knowledge of Economic Development in the West Midlands was encyclopedic. Realizing that we were all worried about handing in our first essay she gave us extensive guidance the most memorable of which was her explanation of the 'fog index'. In Barbara's opinion most students tried to use sentences that were overly long to express their academic ideas. Barbara's fog index' was a rule that if a sentence was over twelve words long it could be split into shorter sentences to intensify the focus and clarity of a students expression. She particularly tried to discourage students from using sentences that were a paragraph long. She also argued that computer spell checks were not a substitute for the discipline of proof reading (something I should have taken to heart I feel).

Going to Barbara's lectures for the first time I felt very insecure and found a need to participate in every debate. A regular sparring partner was Desmond, an overseas student from Jamaica who had very strong Thatcherite views. Desmond's place on the course was paid for by the Jamaican government to which he would return once he had completed the course. Much of the opportunity to contribute in debates and receive essays back (which were clearly way above the pass mark for Postgraduate Diploma level) boosted my confidence. Ultimately what made the difference was the ability to transfer to Masters level at the end of my first year.

A major obstacle to achieving at Masters level was the need to take summer examinations for the Economic Development part of the course. Juggling part time hours of study with a full time job was difficult and I could just about manage to hand in essays which though well written out were poorly proof read. I decided to discuss the issue with my tutor Gill Bently. I told her those three weeks after my last examination I had had a nervous breakdown. She told me that she would go to the Faculty Board and discuss what I had said. After a week or so Gill fed back to me what they had decided.
The good news was that I would not have to take any examinations. However, the bad news was that I would have two assignments, both of three thousand words in addition to the mandatory five thousand extended essays everybody completed.

These pieces of work would have to be completed in six weeks. At the same time I was being bullied at work and decided the best way of coping was to talk to my doctor. She recommended three weeks of sick leave which coincided with this period of essay writing. Fortunately, I met the deadlines for the work and finished the year on an average mark of sixty-eight percent which was well above the sixty percent required for a transfer to Masters from Postgraduate Diploma.

Gill Bentley taught the Economic Development module after Chris Collinge had had to focus on delivering a departmental research project to a tight deadline. Much of the course focused on the localized effects of 'Globalization' the movement away from a mass production, mass consumption society. This society was replaced by one where companies focused on niche markets, 'just in time' production methods and the contracting out of peripheral activities. That may sound like rocket science but the effect of all the above trends was to make many jobs short term and insecure whilst the ultimate threat was that jobs could be shifted to countries where labour costs were more competitive. Many of our case studies concentrated on activities of local councils (such as Sheffield and London) in trying to generate local jobs through inward investment. The first year of the course was delivered in the year that preceded the 1997 General Election. A topical book of the time was written by Will Hutton and entitled 'The State We're In'. This book was essentially a critique of the Thatcher-Major era and was recommended to me by Barbara.

My Second Year.

To get a Masters degree I had to sustain a mark of over sixty percent in the research module and in the remaining dissertation.

The statistics and quantitative methods course seemed straight forward but I just scrapped through on a sixty percent pass in the assignment. I found much of the coursework familiar and missed the occasional lecture. The lecture I missed covered the important areas on reflection such as the philosophy of research including questions such as what is reality. These were areas I would have to cover in my research thesis a couple of years later.

The next research methods course was entitled qualitative methods and caught my imagination. The course was delivered in a challenging way by Moyra Riseborough and highlighted the array of different methods that could be used and the contrasting sociological perspectives that underpinned them. It was a struggle to understand the theory. We were given a useful assignment to critically appraise a piece of published research. On the advice of Dr. Marian Barnes (later to become a professor and my research supervisor) I read a book of published research entitled 'Parenting Under Pressure' by

Tim and Wendy Booth. This was a book about how some service users with a learning disability were supported to maintain a role as a parent. I tried to understand how people with learning disabilities would construct their own reality as a means of appraising the research methods used. I got a very high mark for the work.

In my second qualitative methods assignment I used ethno-graphic research methods to analyse the use of space in a residential care setting for mental health service users. When analyzing the diagrams with coded lines drawn on them, I concluded that there were distinctive and contrasting patterns in the way staff and residents used space in the residential home.

For the second piece of work I again got a high mark. Moyra was to supervise me on my dissertation about identifying the barriers that disabled people experience in finding employment.

Moyra was to inspire much of my late thinking on disability by getting me to think about the social model of disability which up until that point in 1997 I had not heard of. She recommended I read a book by Michael Oliver entitled 'The Politics of Disablement'. This book had been written by a disabled person and strikingly had a picture on the cover in which a wheelchair users' path to the polling station was blocked by a flight of stairs.

Michael Oliver wrote about an understanding of disability where disabled people were not so much disabled by the functional impairments (as those who practiced the medical approach had traditionally argued) but by the disabling way in which prejudice, discrimination and the erection of physical, material and political barriers prevent full and active citizenship within society. This may seem a convoluted definition but an example of the social models application helps explain this. A disabled person for example could be someone with a severe hearing impairment in British society. Doctors would blame this persons struggle to communicate on their hearing impairment. However, if this person were to fly to the United States to live among a community there called Martha's Vineyard; their ability to community would improve. This is because a large proportion of the population who live on Martha's Vineyard can use sign language. Even if this sign language were a variant of British Sign Language it would not take long to adapt. This is because sign language is a form of communication developed and owned by deaf people. Sign language was not officially recognized until the early1970's. If people took the time and trouble to learn sign language it is possible that fewer hearing impaired people would struggle to communicate. Therefore, in the social model, a person's impairment does not necessarily lead to disability.

Despite feeling inspired my reading for my dissertation was not broad enough and I relied on as little as twenty sources for my first draft. Problems in proof reading also surfaced and in addition to this the structure of the dissertation was inappropriate. I took away the first draft and redrafted it along the lines recommended and rewrote and proof read. However, without an ideal structure and much extra reading I had underestimated what was required. After receiving the first draft back I was in crisis. It was November 1998 and I had started my registration for an MPhil degree in October. How would I juggle everything? I phoned Professor Anne Davis who said that though this was a difficult time, if I could come through it, it would help me in my long term academic development. I met up with Dr. Marian Barnes (later to become a professor) who read through my dissertation, then wrote six words on a piece of paper to suggest a structure and suggestions of further reading and asked me to go and write up.

In February 1999 I handed in a completely rewritten dissertation (with no further assistance) to Moyra and after minor amendments I had finally got my Masters Degree.

I graduated on July 9th, 1999. This time in contrast to 1987 I was mentally well.

Registering for an MPhil.

At the same time as coming up with the idea for my Masters dissertation I also started to consider whether I could study for a doctorate. I saw Peter Simon in the Centre for Urban and Regional Studies who tried to ensure that I knew what I was letting myself in for. I think I remember him trying to dissuade me. I told him I wanted to explore employment matters for people with mental health issues. He could see I was keen but said I would have to get in touch with the Department of Social Policy and Social Work (as it was then called) and speak to Professor Ann Davis. Professor Ann Davis was on study leave so I went to Marian who suggested I write a research proposal. She made some suggestions for initial reading.

I struggled to write and showed a draft of the research proposal to Peter Fox a neighbour (who worked in the School of Education at the University). He said I had all the ingredients but needed a structure. He suggested a structure (I went away to completely rewrite the proposal) and then I presented it to Marian who said it should be good enough to get first year funding so that I could study for a research degree.

MY RESEARCH DEGREE EXPERIENCE.

I had been accepted as a research student because my research proposal or plan of research had been considered original and realistic in terms of my being able to be carried out. In this plan I wanted to 'Identify the Main Characteristics of Paid Work that could Enable Fellow Mental Health Service Users to Find, retain and thrive in Employment'.

A mental health service user is someone who has been so severely ill at sometime in their life that they have needed to be admitted to a psychiatric hospital. I decided to write about issues of promoting employment for those who had been diagnosed with severe mental health problems because as a mental health user myself I had been discriminated because of my disability.

If you are not interested in the academic research process please feel free to skip a few pages to read of the lessons I learned from my research.

What I was trying to find out.

Part of my approach to the overall research topic outlined above, was to study the relationship between an individual mental health service user's well-being and nine characteristics of their work environment in their most recent or present job. These job characteristics were very complex but some of these were factors such as task variety, degree of autonomy at work, level of pay, opportunity to socially interact and so on.

The research methods I used to help me find out this information were a survey (or survey method) where I used self completion questionnaires.
In another part of the research topic it was more important to understand aspects of mental health service user's experiences of employment and illness contextualized within their unique life

journeys. The understanding of such experiences was important to piece together important themes relevant to the issues of employment and mental health but which are too complex to capture in a questionnaire. In this part of the research project I carried out semi-structured interviews with twenty mental health service users. This type of interview is carried out using a list of important topics by me as the researcher with each person I interviewed.

It is difficult to summaries what I was trying to find out briefly. Broadly I was trying to find out what worked for mental health service users in employment and what did not. More specifically I probed interviewees about types of supervision and support (lack of support) they received, as well as the disabling/ enabling social and physical work environments in which they were located.
I also used a specifically constructed topic guide to interview ten employer/ support organizations that had had experience of working with mental health service users.

How I analysed the information gathered.

When analysing the information from the interview I split my findings into two chapters of my research thesis. Firstly, I wrote one chapter by identifying themes from individual typed records of individual interviews (called transcripts). The transcripts were hundreds of pages long altogether. Each interview was about 15 pages long on average which meant that there were nearly 450 pages of transcripts. I split the transcripts into negative and positive themes or issues which were then summarized with extracts from the transcripts to illustrate particular points. Secondly, I analysed each transcript individually to examine how key individuals had made sense of their experiences in similar, related and contrasting ways. For me the way mental health service users made sense of their experience (or constructed their own sense of meaning from experience) was valuable and crucial to the whole research project.

I also analysed the questionnaires from the survey to statistically measure the strength of relationships between how mental health service users perceived the quality of their present or last work environment with their perception of the quality of their own mental health.

Lessons I learned from my research.

I have consigned the period of study for research degree as a difficult experience which I an only partially re-visiting with the writing of this chapter. The truth is I do not have the heart to read over the thesis which symbolizes so much labour of love/ hate for me. For those who want to pour over the details for themselves I am reliably informed there is a reference copy of my thesis in Birmingham University Library.

I have no wish to quote the research findings in a way that would be the protocol of an academic article. For my findings to be accurately quoted for academic purposes my thesis needs to be read, accurately quoted and referenced correctly. For the purposes of my autobiography I am giving a very abridged version of what I learned from my research.

An important lesson for me was that most mental health service users have experience of employment even if this is a short and negative one. Most people assume that because someone is diagnosed with a mental health problem that they have no experience of work. This in my opinion is wrong.

My feeling, after the project had been going for two years, was that I was working with mental health service users whose experience came under two broad categories. Firstly, there are those who have had a bad experience/s of work which they feel has contributed to their low self esteem or to their mental illness. For these people, receipt of disability benefit, attending a day centre or attending a sheltered employment workshop seemed the best option or what worked for them.

Secondly, there are those people who have had poor experiences of work and seemed able to move on to better employers with whom most of them were still employed. Many of these people seemed able to get help form a specialist employment agency or job broker to sell their skills first to an employer before talking about accommodations for their disability. Often these people were able to get benefits check to see whether or not they would lose out financially by taking a job. Often specialist job agencies were valued because they built confidence and prevented mental health service users from undervaluing their skills. Many of these mental health service users interviewed were employed by voluntary or statutory sectors of the mental health system. It is these employers who have started to realize the real asset of lived experience of mental health distress that can enable their services to be more relevant to their client's needs.

The challenge of research.

Whilst carrying out and transcribing my interviews with fellow mental health survivors, an unexpected interview topic emerged. Some survivors had mentioned that when attempting to manage their mental health through difficult periods in their life they had encountered suicidal feelings. Reflection in these interviews and interview transcripts was difficult because I was revisiting emotional issues that had caused my first breakdown at the time. However, with the help of a friend called Fiona I was able to get through this tricky period.

Analysing over 400 pages of interview transcripts and splitting the interviews into segments that corresponded with different themes was challenging. However, as the themes began to emerge from my analysis it felt like the whole research project was beginning to emerge like the completion of a giant jigsaw puzzle. This experience of research analysis was one of the most exhilarating experiences of my academic life. The chapter of findings based on my analysis seemed to write itself because everything came together so nicely.

In the autumn of 2002 I had enrolled on the Postgraduate Diploma in Social Work course at Birmingham University. I attended 20-25 hours of lectures per week in addition to the course requirements of handing in two assignments. I still had to find, in addition to this, ten hours a week for writing my research thesis. I was also working in a residential unit for mental health service users 18.5 hours per week and fulfilling a role as student mentor at Jarratt Hall one evening a week. I was still putting the final touches to my thesis with all these impossible demands. In practice I just wanted to complete my thesis with the minimum required effort. Professor Ann Davis made some suggestion for final writing up. I typed up her suggestions diligently but did not proof read afterwards. A partial reason for this was the fact that I was ill without openly acknowledging it to myself and furthermore I was trying to work under feelings of extreme fatigue. In January 2003, a month before my oral exam or viva, I went to the doctor for a check up and discovered I had blood pressure readings that caused the practice nurse and Dr. Cross some concern. Dr. Cross was sufficiently concerned to lend me an electronic blood pressure reading machine under strict orders to take three readings for a fortnight.

After submitting the thesis in November 2002 I finally found the energy to read it and immediately realized I had handed in a piece of work that was to some extent flawed. I was worried about my viva and phoned professor Ann Davis numerous times who said that in her opinion I would probably have to make amendments and that I should not worry too much because in her opinion the worst case scenario was that I would get an MPhil, a lower, but still reputable degree. However she said it probably would not come to that. Marian Barnes (now a newly appointed professor of Social Research) told me not to worry about any perceived thoughts I had about faults in my thesis. She said that in her opinion what you could not take away from my research was an original contribution to existing knowledge.

The climax of the research experience – my viva.

I had asked to be excused from lectures on the day of February 25th, 2003, my viva and had spent most of the morning walking around campus and talking to various academic staff. I realized that this was one of the most important days of my life in which honest judgment would be passed on passed on four years of my life's commitment to research and indirectly on my level academic achievement to this point.

Before meeting my examiners I met my supervisors. Professor Ann Davis said before I went in, that judgment by academic peers could be delivered in such a way that it was difficult not to take it personally.

The examiners had allowed one of my supervisors, Professor Marian Barnes to sit in. Then the examiners Professor Barratt (my internal examiner) and Dr. Wetherspoon (my external examiner) walked in with the independent invigilator Dr. Mike Nellis. After greetings and shaking of hands all round proceedings were underway.

Dr. Wetherspoon fed back straight away by saying that the thesis was an impressive, monumental and original piece of research. However, he said that it did not reach doctorate standard. My heart sank but I knew I had to remain focused. There was then some discussion about immediate feedback without a proper viva. Nevertheless, in the end the viva went ahead.

According to the examiners there were inconsistencies in my approach to the research aims, questions and research strategy. I managed to keep my nerve, my cool and my temper by explaining how my research had evolved. I painstakingly justified every single decision I had made about the research which was an excellent verbal response. My reply about my evolving approach was according to the examiners not sufficiently signposted in the thesis itself. Specifically, Professor Barratt felt that there were insufficient introductions and conclusions to the chapters in my thesis to guide the reader through my evolving development of literature and the research process itself. There were also problems with the referencing and missing pages to the thesis.

Dr. Wetherspoon then angrily told me that it was clear I had not proof read my thesis. What he did not realize was that I was angry with the way he had pulled my thesis apart without any detailed positives about what I had tried to achieve.

He then said 'I kept coming across sentences with missing words'. As a way of shielding myself from the pain and anger I started humming 'Missing Words' from the band called the selector (an early 1980's Ska group) to myself to blot out any more wounding criticism.

After a fifteen minute recess both my supervisors and I were called back to get the final feedback. It was clear from the feedback that, particularly from the independent invigilator Dr. Mike Nellis, that I had given a good verbal performance and from what they were saying they wanted to give me a further chance to prove myself. I feel they were so impressed that I seemed to know what I was talking about that they felt they still wanted to leave the door open for me to revise and resubmit for a doctorate. However, the devastating news was that a substantial revision was still required to attain an MPhil.

I cried shortly after the feedback. People asked me how I felt at the time and I said 'Like I just flushed four years of my life down the toilet'. Professor Ann Davis was quick to remind me that the then head of our department was qualified to MPhil standard. Marian said however that failure to get a doctorate was a setback if I wanted to pursue an academic career.

However, I still wanted to resubmit for a doctorate as well as juggling a social work course. Professor Ann Davis gave me a stern reality check on that option a few weeks later and I chose somewhat reluctantly to resubmit for an MPhil.

Picking up the pieces.

When I agonized and then progressed in the rewriting progress I needed friends with whom I could talk social research jargon. My main support came from fellow research students Tula and Nicki and occasionally a lecturer called Guy. It was amazing how many jargon word I fitted in with my short meetings with these people. I am grateful to them for all being there as my academic peers through this difficult period.

To start the whole resubmission process off, Professor Marian Barnes consulted Professor Barratt to get a summary of the nature of re-writing what was needed to attain an MPhil degree. Marian then gave a few written pages of instructions and I was asked to go away and completely re-write the thesis before resubmitting it for any more supervision.

To make time to re-write my thesis, juggle my social work course and finish both at the time in synchronization with other students on the course.

I had to delay my second social work placement by six months and then I had a fraction of the time of everyone else to hand in my last five thousand word assignment.

I had to understand Marian's instructions if I were to get through and reading it through it all seemed too much. I lay in bed depressed for ages and wanted to give up. I kept thinking of how I could broach it to Marian. But I knew that neither Marian nor Ann would accept my resignation now no matter how persuasively I felt I was able to put the case at the time.

When I finally had the heart to pick up my thesis and read it again Marian's instructions started to make sense and I started to piece things together bit-by-bit. Things went well until chapter five when I ran out of steam. Out of frustration I left a few messages for Professor Ann Davis in the early hours of the morning when I had finished my work for the day, only to be woken up when she called me at 8am in the morning. I answered the call yawning and then slept for another hour.

I then met with my final supervision session with Marian who commented on my main strength to get to the verge of getting my MPhil was my staying power. She said her recent advice to prospective research students was that they needed staying power - 'You've certainly got that' she said.

Both Ann and Marian read through my resubmitted thesis. Ann stated about a week later that work still needed to be done but on the whole she was uplifted by the improvement in my writing style. I then resubmitted my thesis to find to my dismay that there were still missing pages. Despite that the examiners were prepared to award an MPhil subject to minor amendments. Ann told me sternly that I would need to get it right next time if I were to graduate in the summer.

Fortunately I graduated (in the presence of my wife, brother, the Anglican Chaplain Alistair, lecturers Dr. Jan Waterson and Gill Bentley) but was disappointed that nine out of ten chapters of my thesis were of doctorate standard. So close and yet so very far.

Three years on from my oral examination or viva, I am very grateful that I did come out with something to show for the huge amount of debt incurred whilst I was a student. With academic qualifications, professional contract research and lecturing experience as well as a professional qualification and registration with a professional body, I have the developed potential to have made my employment situation more secure.

The experience of having to juggle many competing priorities as a student has prepared me well for the pressure of social work. My experience of disability and the real nature of prejudice and discrimination in the real world out there has made me even more determined to succeed. Meanwhile, I have to realize that I am lucky compared to most people with a similar disability, which makes me realize that I have to try and appreciate what I have done and savour some of the relative power, status and privilege that I have. I am always conscious that I must not take my mental well being for granted. I have a higher risk of developing clinical illness than most other people. Looking at the worst case scenario, if I were to become severely unwell again and I lost my job, I could still look at the period between my second and third nervous breakdowns with pride and no one can take that away from me.

CHAPTER NINE.

BECOMING A SOCIAL WORKER.

Early notions of social work.

I was often perceived by myself and my foster mother as being a bit scatter brained. I did not seem able to get my head around anything practical without forgetting to do something important.

The idea I had about social work then was mainly related to Dr. Mason who had been the nearest thing to a practitioner I had seen in my childhood. Social work was this messy complex thing I could not understand or hope to get a grip of.

It was not until I was to encounter episodes of mental health problems in the 1980's that I thought seriously about the nature of the social work role in any length. When I was in hospital after experiencing my second nervous breakdown there was a nursing assistant called Sian. I had told her I had a degree and that I wanted to put something back into the mental health care system that had provided for me. She then said something amazing to me knowing that I had a diagnosis of a severe mental health problem. 'Why don't you try and become a social worker?' I was shocked by what she had said knowing full well the experience I had had of discrimination in the job market. I also doubted whether I could get funding to study again after already having had one bite at the cherry. However, without realizing it at the time she had sown a seed in my head. I always wondered what she saw in me that suggested I would be a suitable social worker.

However, by this time I also realized there was such a thing as a mental health social worker and I was fascinated by the way they had helped me. There was a hospital social worker who played a big role in liaising with my employer while I was ill in hospital and negotiating a phased introduction to work as I got better.

My first community mental health social worker was Gill. She said to me that I was one of her first clients. She was young and had just graduated from Birmingham University. Over a number of months she was my advocate in a tricky situation around my benefits after leaving a postal filing clerk job I no longer felt able to do. She then initiated some work (finished off by a social work assistant, Sharon) to find me housing where I could live independently with my wife in the community. She spent an initial session with me just asking questions which I later learned was an assessment. Essentially Gill and Sharon had together enabled me to move on from my illness to the next phase of my life.

An introduction to the social model of disability.

In 1997 I was introduced to a book that enabled me to understand how social workers had started to think about disability. In my first session with my dissertation supervisor, Moyra. I was asked whether I had ever heard of a book called 'The Politics of disablement' by Michael Oliver. I said I had   not and followed up on her suggestion.

What I discovered on reading this book was an understanding of disability from the perspective of some disabled people who had become academics. I understood that providing enabling environments for people was key.   I also understood that focusing on people's strengths rather than their disabilities was a way of maximizing a person's potential for independence.

This book was crucial in enabling me to build a social model understanding of mental illness. It forced me to look at my own disability in a different way. Rather than blaming things that I could not do on my illness I began to look at my strengths. This was a period in my life when I had the audacity to plan to do a doctorate. I felt that I could liberate other mental health service users from negative understandings of their disability through my research and practical work.

Whilst I was doing my doctorate I developed and appreciation by lecturing student mental health social workers on the importance of the social model of disability in social work and the formation of social work values.

The power of the profession discourse.

Whilst I was working for Rethink in a rehabilitation unit for people with mental health problems I found

I developed a professional key worker relationship with up to four residents. I often arranged reviews where social workers were invited. Social workers sometimes expressed professional views which were at odds with my own assessment of the situation. The social workers did not know the residents anywhere near as much as I did and often the resident's views were overridden as well. The review often ended with the professional view prevailing over anything that the key worker or resident thought. It was at this stage I understood how professional understandings of disability were far more powerful than the understandings disabled people had of their own disability or that of unqualified staff who worked with them on a daily basis.

I particularly understood how the medical understanding of mental health issues was particularly powerful and often articulated by the psychiatrist at the review. I felt that the only person with any sort of power to challenge the medical understanding of the psychiatrist was the social worker.

My appointment with the careers advisor.

It was December 2001 and my final year of writing up my thesis. During this time I had come to a realization that an academic career was a distant hope. Most of the jobs in research were short term contracts. A job as a lecturer seemed a difficult prospect because I was not clear that I had a specialist area of knowledge and expertise where I could fit into the vacancies I saw advertised in University departments across the country. Furthermore, I might well end up working in another part of the country which would mean that I would not be able to keep my commitment of caring for my wife and brother.

I decided around 10th/11th December 2001 around two weeks before Christmas to visit the University careers service on campus. I met up with someone who asked me my purpose in coming. I explained my situation of writing up my thesis and feeling that I could not find an academic career. He asked me what I was good at. I replied that I was a bit of a people person really. He then sarcastically said 'In that case why don't you try working as a mortuary attendant?' He was trying to tell me to be more specific. I explained that I was good at working with people who had very low self esteem to allow them to see themselves more positively and I was good at motivating people. I was good at listening to people but not only listening but actively listening and reflecting back to them what they had said to me in a way that made them feel understood. He asked if I had considered a career in social work or the probation service. I told him that social work appealed but that I would not get funding because of local authority funding for my previous degree. It was explained to me that I could get funding for a postgraduate qualification in social work but if I wanted to get on that years intake I needed to get my application in within days.

I remember feeling that this was not the first time that someone had suggested a career in social work and felt in a curious way that it was my fate but an acceptable and suitable fate for me. Every time there seemed to be an obstacle in my way in terms of finances and arrangements about finishing off my thesis the problem was overcome. Fate indeed.

I had a useful conversation with Professor Ann Davis about how things could be juggled so I could finish off my thesis when I started on the social work course. She felt that becoming a social work student would potentially damage my ability to do my thesis and impede my progress as a social work student. In the end she was proved partially right, my thesis did suffer. However, in my head I had to an extent already given up on an academic career so perhaps my thesis was not as important. However I did not feel that my thesis would suffer at the time and was not aware of the nature of the academic sacrifice I was to eventually make.

Being a social work student: Attending lectures and writing assignments.

I am not sure as I gained as much from my experience as a social work student as I would have liked. Most of the lectures were crammed into the first five months of my first year which made the course seem top heavy. Much of the theory around social work was structured in courses that explored themes about identity and social structure, human development, diverse communities, social work theories and models and social work social skills. To have gained more from the course I feel I should have read more widely rather than just preparing material for written assignments. Because some of my attention was centered on completing my thesis I did not have adequate time to reflect on what had been taught. The whole experience was overwhelming physically as well as mentally and by the time our first phase of lectures was drawing to a close in February 2003 I was diagnosed with borderline high blood pressure which meant daily monitoring using a machine on loan from my doctor.

It did not mean the lectures weren't interesting but I was struggling to maintain concentration through physical exhaustion. I had to complain about the very abrasive style of one children's law lecturer at one stage as I felt he was making me physically ill.

Emma and Vicky were good at making me relax and they suggested bringing in some snacks to break up the day and to take a toilet break if things got too much. Emma was a long-term friend I made while I was a student. She always seemed to find the funny side of things and helped me from taking life too seriously when I was going through a stressful time.

One of the very difficult projects I had to undertake as a student was community profiling. My assignment was to understand the needs of the Irish Community in Selly Oak. After studying maps detailing the distribution of the Irish community in Birmingham as a whole one issue became very apparent. You may need to think outside of the box when meeting an individual's cultural needs.

The Irish community in the south of Birmingham was mainly centered around Digbeth, parts of Balsall Heath and Moseley. To get an understanding involved firstly studying the history of Irish settlers in Britain in the Industrial Revolution and after the Second World War. Understanding the history of Irish people in Britain led me to study the history of Irish people in Birmingham. I understood that many of the potential resources to support the Irish community in Selly Oak were based in Digbeth. The object of the exercise was to understand that any of the service users we came into contact with could come from any ethnic group in potentially any part of the city. The assignment taught me to seek resources outside a person's immediate neighbourhood to meet their needs. It was also a warning that when a person's ethnic group forms such a small part of the community their potential cultural needs can be overlooked.

Much of the material around racial identity and awareness was taught on a CD Rom. However, Tarsem who coordinated part of this course wanted to stir up a debate around issues of race and ethnicity. I could honestly see his point. There are some students who feel the best way to get through a social work course is not necessarily to be honest about their values. Some people will sit silently in lectures and trot out what they think the markers want to read in their assignments. For these people, the student experience is not as transformative as it could be leaving racist, oppressive views that a student holds unchallenged. I always ensured that I made a contribution to the debate in lectures knowing full well that my views could be challenged but knowing that in exposing myself to that risk I was also exposing myself to a new leaning opportunity. Tarsem and I were able to challenge each other and both of us learned something new from participating in debates on the issues around race and ethnicity.

The human development lectures were my favourite because of the spice to the subject added by the lecturer Richard Downey. I attended lectures around child development and the importance of attachment theory. However my interest was focused on adolescent development and how mature and older adults dealt with change later in their lives. Richard did a particularly good lecture on mid-life crisis and how humans come to terms with their own mortality. His humour was brilliant. He told the story of being a fan of the 1950's cowboy series 'Rawhide' to such an extent that he tried to track down horses in the middle of inner city Liverpool as a child.

Much of the social work law in my first year was taught in a way in which you were encouraged not necessarily to know what the law was but to know how to go about finding out relevant legislation, case law and government guidance if presented with practical examples of a problem in our the course of our future work. The two law assignments we had to complete were around practical examples we could find in our first placement. In my first placement I worked with a service user with a learning disability whom I suspected was being financially abused by parents. In my second placement I examined the community care legislation, case law and government guidance relevant to an older adult living in the community.

When examining issues around social identity and structure I tried to explore in my assignment the continuing relevance of class in an essay on the underclass. According to Roy Hattersley, in a classic *Guardian* End piece article, those with wealth and capital are able to continue to pass on their advantage to their children. Because of this, class and its accompanying inequality is, in my opinion, still as relevant as ever. Tony Blair's endeavour to create a society where there is 'equality of opportunity' does not deal with the fundamental causes of the inequality in this country because those from more privileged backgrounds are better able to exploit those opportunities. Hattesley's views echo my own.

It is easy to argue that the class analysis of Marx is redundant. Marxism is to some extent no longer relevant to a world where the relationship between capital and labour has evolved to a more complex distinction than that of the contemporary mid-19th Century world of Marx himself.

However, Neo-Marxists have taken into account the changes in the nature of capitalism and make many more distinctions in the types of bourgeoise (or owners of capital). They make distinctions between institutional ownership of capital, individual shareowners and landowners and people who are directors or managers who exert power over workers but have no ownership or capital. There is now international or global ownership of some capital which means workers can be made to accept particular working conditions or face a whole shift of capital (the production plant) to another country. Because trade unions have failed to become international in response to the global organisation of capital there is a limit in the ability working class movements such as trade unions to negotiate concessions which may address inequalities in the distribution of income from wealth in society. Therefore, equalities in the ownership of land and capital, plus inability to negotiate an ethical distribution of the revenue of what we sell, lie at the heart of inequality in any industrialized society.

It is almost universally recognized in academic literature that inequalities in income lead to inequalities in health. As there is greater incidence of health problems amongst those defined by a lower socio-economic status in each population census and this leads to these people needing proportionately more social care. Yet those with better education are more likely, in my limited experience as a social worker, to understand their rights and to be able to consume proportionately more social care services as a result. I strongly feel that there is an inequality in the distribution of finite social care services. People who struggle with the English language or who are poorly educated or inarticulate are less likely to know their rights and are probably not going to receive what the law says they are entitled to.

After the experience of being a social work student you never really listen to ordinary conversation in the same way again. The more I gained experience of academic life the more I understood the importance of language in the formations of ideas and more importantly, attitudes. In appropriate attitudes which are part of poor sets of values lead to vulnerable groups in society being poorly treated, denied their human rights and being stereotyped or prejudged by those who have not taken the trouble to know them as individuals at all. Vulnerable people can have power exerted over them by those charged with their care. Being aware of the differences in power in sets of relationships is an important part of the social work role. Failure to challenge discrimination, language, stereotypes and oppressive behaviour often leads to people, who lack power in a given relationship, to experience an intrusion on their human rights. As one lecturer said 'if you are not part of the solution, you are part of the problem'. Inaction is a form of collusion with those who oppress others. There are those who feel that being challenged in their use of language is an affront. These people often feel that those who challenge are part of an agenda of political correctness prevalent in society today. However, if people have come to think about how they refer to others then this is a much needed form of consideration for others that can only lead to less powerful people being treated better in society in the long run.

I feel that because I completed assignments to pass the course, rather than to maximize my learning opportunities, I missed out on a more thorough understanding of the social work role. Assignments are an exciting learning experience if you have the necessary time, energy and health to really do them justice. I wish on reflection I had had the opportunity to focus single mindedly on social work training. However, my decision to spread myself thinly and ration my exertion of energy was an effective survival strategy that led me to complete the course without any severe health problems.

Philip Hill

My Practice Placements.

My first placement was with a learning disabilities team that provided service users with opportunities to access the community for education, training, employment, travel and leisure experiences. The local authority had a vision that people with learning disabilities should access the community for their day activities and therefore be seen as valued citizens. In reality all the work should have involved a worker doing assessments in people's homes and then working with them through a period of transition in which they became used to a routine around their day activities. However, the place from which I worked was in effect a drop-in centre for service users who still seemed to regard it as a form of day centre.
The problem with most placements is that they struggle to find students sufficient activities. My supervisor Alyson was aware of this and tried very hard to talk to colleagues to set up a sufficient variety of work to meet what were then called competences.

I was aware from day one that all the service users I was working with were adults. What angered me was that some carers still treated their sons and daughters as children. What horrified me was the extent to which money which belonged to service users was put in the family pot with them having to ask permission for small amounts of pocket money. I immediately felt there were issues with many service users not leading the independent lives they were capable of because they had never been given the opportunity to make important decisions over their lives. Risk assessments could often be used to deny service user's important experiences that non disabled people take for granted. Then I understood that there were two types of learning disability, one was medically defined and the other an absence of opportunities to learn because of the service users being surrounded by people over protecting them. Whilst there is a need to protect vulnerable adults, a more person centred approach to risk assessment would enable service users to experience richer lives from which they could learn more.

I went on an exhilarating training day in which I understood that people with learning disabilities without communication skills could communicate very complex things to carers through an imaginative use of everyday objects being attached to touching mechanisms. This was a very good way in which service users could express choice. For example, a comb could be attached to one switch and a chocolate wrapper to another leaving it open to a service user to express that choice by touching that object.

I also watched an excellent People First presentation in which they asked us in the audience to explain the meaning of commonly used 'hard words'. I also watched them present a play in which they explained how people with learning disabilities were discriminated against and excluded because much of the information commonly available in society were written using 'hard words' whilst at the same time failing to use plain English.

I learned about a type of person centred planning called 'Gifts and Skills'. Using a mixture of writing and images I helped service users identify positive things about themselves as well as drawing attention to strengths or 'gifts' that they or their circle of support thought they possessed. Only those invited by the service user made up their circle of support.

I found that the quality of my learning experience on my first placement was good but that the qualities of learning opportunities were not sufficient to the extent that I was using a small range of learning experiences to meet a lot of my competencies. I found however that I had discovered one service user group that I wanted to work with.

My second placement was initially based in the Appointee and Receivership Section. Working alongside Sheila and her colleagues gave me insights into issues of mental capacity which I had struggled with since finishing my first placement. I had to revisit issues around what is mental capacity and who is able to assess this (and on what criteria they made a capacity decision). I also gained a firmer grasp of what financial abuse was by studying some old referrals to the team. I was also given the opportunity to write letters to GP's, the Department of Works and Pensions and carers. However, because this placement did not give me sufficient opportunities to meet service users, John (my long arm supervisor) organized a further placement with and older adult's team.

My practice teacher Mir gave me a huge number of learning opportunities and soon my caseload built steadily to six cases. When it came to doing my competency document I had so much evidence I could afford to exclude some of it and choose the best examples of how I had met a particular competence. I discovered very quickly that I did not want to work with this client group because I identified very heavily with the difficult transitions that those going into residential care had to make and could visualize myself occupying the same space forty years down the road. What particularly hit home to me was someone who went into residential care and had previously been a social worker. As one lecturer said to me 'Ageism is the only 'ism' that gets its revenge'.

During my second placement I took a day out to visit the Social Care Jobs Fair at the International Convention Centre. I went to the Birmingham stand and met up with Liz Wakeley. When I explained a bit about my experience she gave me strong advice to apply immediately for Social Work posts that had just been advertised in 'The Voice' even though I did not qualify until six months later.

I was to meet Liz again at the interview along with my current manager Bethan. I decided the best strategy to keep a lid on the nerves was to say to myself that I probably would not get the job and that I could still rely on myself to get agency work. My preparation was a day out in Cambridge in which on the long train journey I managed to cram in eight hours preparation. I managed to keep my composure and after the first five minutes I felt comfortable. The questions ranged from easy (what so you think makes a good assessment?) to hard (how would I assess someone without verbal communication skills?) I felt I was getting good vibes but was not sure until the end of the interview when Liz said she had enjoyed interviewing me. It took them less than 90 minutes and Liz left a message on my phone saying I had got the job.

I had got a job in the social work field that, as a child I had always thought was too complicated for me. The academic door had been well and truly shut but at the same time the social work door had opened very widely indeed.

I feel that I have been a learning disabilities social worker for 18-months and yet I have not got sufficient grasp of my role to write anything telling about my experience. Suffice to say I am at a stage where the learning curve is still steep. I did however imagine I would have all this power to transform situations for service users and did not realize how often in my role I would feel powerless.

Footnote : My struggle to become a Registered Social Worker.

There is a requirement for all social workers employed in England and Wales to be registered with the General Social Care Council. There was an initial period in which I did not have to be registered but there was a requirement to have sent off my form and prove that I did 'not intend to deceive'. Therefore, while my registration was being processed I was covered to practice.

In the end it proved an agonizing wait. I left it four months and phoned up only to be told they had only just entered my details on the system. A month later I was told that my application would take at least another six months to process because there had been a declaration on the health part of the form.

By this time I was beginning to feel a bit insecure and I had a right to be. Nine months after submitting my application form for registration I was sent a self assessment form to fill in. What was quite clear from the phrasing of the questions was that not only was there a need to relate my experience of my illness honestly but that there were some definite right and wrong answers to the questions about my professional approach to service users and carers. I was pretty quick to point to the overarching guidelines of the General Social Care Council as a means of a reference point for my practice. I also pointed out that if I had managed two full time courses at University and a part time job then I might be able to manage 36 hours of being a full time social worker. I was pretty angered that a body such as the General Social Care Council should use such oppressive questions to refer to my disability, such as how do you manage your condition? My answer to this was that I regarded my illness of Schizophrenia by a less oppressive term of a mental health issue, terminology which I then used throughout my form. The good thing about this form was a question about how managers support you at work.

I was to find yet again that my psychiatrist was to be a gatekeeper to any opportunities that I could access and his timely written response as a medical referee was a giant piece of the jigsaw that needed to be completed. Finally, I had to seek access to the notes kept on me by the Occupational Health Section of the City Council (with whom I had two medical interviews before I was appointed). It was only when this favourable report was sent that I received a phone call at work at the beginning of October, 2005 stating that the only barriers to registration were now bureaucratic. After nearly a year of waiting I was finally able to access my name onto the General Council website as a registered social worker.

I was to find that disabled people had been discriminated against in the application process because their applications had been singled out as more difficult to assess and left deliberately to later assess as a way of managing the 20.000 or so that arrived in the deadline for registration on December 1st, 2004.

I was right to be worried about my registration because within weeks of getting my registration an Approved Social Worker with mental health issues found he could only register with conditions attached. In addition to this another Social Worker with mental health issues was refused to be registered by the General Social Care Council and later this decision was overturned by an appeals body because the Council had not weighed up all the evidence, most of it favourable, appropriately.

CONCLUSION.

How I feel after writing this book.

Initially, the purpose of writing this book has been to make sense of the change, traumas, disappointments and achievements of the last ten years. Reaching the milestone of my 40th birthday has led me to look back on my life a great deal. After I had written my first draft I then became aware of the potential for my book to have a positive impact amongst mental health survivors and mental health professionals in countering descriptions of mental health service users in terms of medical labels.

After writing the final draft of my autobiography I am aware of a number of psychological processes that have taken place. Firstly I am beginning finally to value myself as a social worker. Secondly I really do feel I have moved on to some extent because I feel valued and supported by colleagues more now than at any time when I was a student. Furthermore, I feel I am being given opportunities within a supportive environment to develop and grow. This is enabling me to move on from the disappointment of not being able to pursue an academic career. A recent visit to a graduation party made me realize that I am now in a better place now than when I was at University. I feel a greater sense of belonging to a social work team than I ever did to an academic community. When I was a research student I always felt so insecure and during that phase of my life I was struggling with issues in my personal life. Overall I felt that being a research student was a very lonely experience. I now feel valued as part of a team and long periods of lonely study are now replaced with hard work interspersed with informal office banter.

I need other people to remind me and sometimes remind myself that I am an intelligent, skilled practitioner with a lot to give to others. Those who have read my autobiography are surprised that I am not more confident and sure in my own sense of judgement. I live with an overriding fear of oppressing people through the clumsy use of power. However, a manager reminded me recently that in her opinion I could not oppress anybody even if I tried!

I have not moved on completely however. Walking around the campus on graduation day recently was still difficult for me and I find it difficult to even look at someone in a Doctoral gown. The lasting legacy of my period as a student is the amount of debt I got myself into. Though I am constantly reminded of the rewards and privileges that go with my educational attainment, I am still mindful of the costs it will take me five years to repay.

My overriding hope for the future is that I am able to build on what I have now and be able to 'fully' apply my education in the service of disadvantaged groups in society. When I consider the mundane and low paid jobs that many people have, with little chance of personal development, then I do feel privileged that over the last ten years I have been nurtured in various demanding roles from Senior Care Officer to Research Student to Social Worker.

I find it difficult to come to terms with the amount of power I have as a social worker. With power comes the responsibility to reflect adequately on my practice so that I am fully able to justify to myself and others the decisions I have made. I have come to a stage in my life where my opinion (albeit based on a sound value and knowledge base) does matter. This comes full circle from oppressive phases of my life when I have known what it is like to have my opinions ignored or suppressed. My reluctance to exert my power as a social worker is related to my own experiences of oppression. However, my role is to uphold the welfare, rights, choices and independence of service users which means that I may have to be quite assertive with carers, other professionals and even my managers to fulfill this role.

I am beginning to look back on my time as an undergraduate more positively. This is because I can finally understand how my experience at Leicester University has made a powerful contribution to where I am now. Before my breakdown in the summer of 1987 I had grown very substantially socially, psychologically and academically over the preceding two and a half years. The problem that I have had over the past 19 years is to perceive my experience at Leicester in terms of how it all ended rather than acknowledging the real growth that took place before my crisis.

When I attended my graduation ceremony in July 1987 it was clear that much of the academic ability had been lost. Furthermore, in the months that followed it was difficult to respond to news of how my peers were doing when I was not only unemployed but unemployable. As a result I lost touch with all my friends. I have recently felt able to re-establish contact with the alumni office at Leicester University and been able to explain how I am doing without saying exclusively that I am a mental health service user.

It took me ten years to get over the negative aspects of the University experience. I met Janet on a commuter train in south London in 1999. I managed to compose myself sufficiently to avoid making a fool of myself and she was able to see that I was okay and studying for a doctorate. Like many people from my distant past she had trouble recognizing me because of the amount of weight I have put on.

I am grateful over the years for the emotional support of family and friends. A big thank you is necessary for my psychiatrist, Professor Femi Oyebode, who actually listened to me when I said

I was overmedicated and has written countless references to key employers, occupational health departments and Birmingham University. In terms of achievements I have not got very far without key gatekeepers giving me opportunities and nurturing my potential. There is not enough space to acknowledge everyone. My foster father was effective in teaching me to read and instilling in me along with my foster mother the need to study and read books. Thanks to my wife for practical and emotion support over the years. Various employers have also taken me on (although it took 300 job applications to get my first chance at a permanent full time post). The disability organization 'Tragic but Brave' were essential in enabling me to believe that my disability could enable me to be an effective professional carer. Gill Bentley, my former tutor, was essential in supporting me through my Masters degree. Finally, Professor Ann Davis and Professor Marian Barnes who gave me the opportunity to develop my potential to become a qualified researcher.

Looking back, I still remember how I felt in the autumn of 1987 when I was discharged from hospital. I did not understand that my academic ability was not lost but merely on deep freeze. One day I would rise from the ashes and not only regain what I had lost but be able to build on it. Looking forward to how I feel now there is a big gap between how people tell me I should feel and how I actually look at my current situation. My recent disappointment in being unable to start an academic career should be put in terms of other achievements of the last 16 years. I say 'should' because people feel I should be proud. I feel however that it is also normal to be ambitious and in these terms the ongoing struggle to move on from something I spent five years dreaming about is entirely understandable. I have never felt that my diagnosis of Schizophrenia should get in the way of maximizing my potential. Without ambition I would not have had the audacity to train as a social worker, to register for a research degree or fund myself through a Master's degree. Without ambition I would not have started a career as a support worker when I was told that people with Schizophrenia cannot work in social care. Without ambition I would still be diagnosed with learning difficulties. As a social worker I want my ambition to fuel the high expectations I have of myself in meeting the choices, needs and aspirations of service users. I want a move away from the normalization mantra in learning disability services. Normal is not always good enough in my view, people's lives should have the potential to be extraordinary, unique and rich in evolving new possibilities.

www.ingramcontent.com/pod-product-compliance
Lightning Source LLC
Chambersburg PA
CBHW031158270326
41931CB00006B/322